BIOHACKS 101

Alekya Bejgam, PhD

DEDICATION

For the dreamers, the doers, the hustlers: May this book fuel your fire and guide you on your journey.

CONTENTS

ACKNOWLEDGMENTS

To my little muse, Arohi—thank you for embracing more mommy-desk-time and fewer playdates with a grace far beyond your years. Your giggles and hugs were my constant reminder of why I wanted to write something meaningful.

To Rohit, my partner in every sense of the word, who picked up the pieces when the house fell apart—literally and figuratively. Your ability to cheer me on, even when the chaos seemed insurmountable, kept my spirits afloat.

To my mother, Rekha, whose meals became the fuel for not just our bodies but my mind. You ensured we didn't starve while I lost myself in drafts and edits. And to my father, Gopal Krishna, who turned into Arohi's yoga guru and walking buddy, giving me the quiet moments I needed to bring this book to life.

To my sister, Priya, your words of encouragement and reminders to keep breaking boundaries echoed in my mind on every tough day. And to my ever-humorous brother-in-law Suraj, thank you for keeping our spirits light and our laughter loud—it's amazing how much a joke can do for the soul.

To my in-laws, Ramadevi and Bagaiah, the unsung heroes of the kitchen, who armed me with instant powders, masalas, and magical mixes that turned cooking into a sprint instead of a marathon. Your thoughtful shortcuts gave me more time to write and less time to worry.

To my incredible friends, thank you for navigating the hustles of new motherhood alongside me, sharing your tricks, and lifting me up when I felt stretched too thin.

And finally, to my big, warm, and endlessly loving extended family—the Ghulekar's, Bejgam's, and Chikatamarla's—you're the backbone of my support system. Thank you for always showing up with love and encouragement in abundance.

This book carries a part of each of you in its pages. Thank you for being my village. 🩶

1 INTRODUCTION

The Chronicles of Generation "Now, Not Later"

Once upon a time, in a world of convenience, dopamine hits, and the eternal glow of screens, lived Generation "Now, Not Later." They were a curious breed—masters of instant gratification, champions of delivery apps, and legends of the "just one more episode" mindset.

The daily routine of most looked something like this:

- **Strength Training:** Regularly lifting their phones to order takeout or scroll social media until their thumbs got stronger than their legs.

- **Endurance:** Binge-watching series with

such commitment that finishing a ten-season show in one weekend became a badge of honor.

- **Flexibility:** Demonstrated in creative excuses to dodge workouts. "Oh, I'd go running, but the humidity is just not right for my vibe today."
- **Cardio:** Sprinting to the fridge during ad breaks.
- **Mental Gymnastics:** Convincing themselves that ordering a salad with the fries balanced out their dietary choices.

The "Next Decade" Mirror

There was an ancient mirror, passed down through generations, said to show the future consequences of today's actions. One brave soul, curious about their trajectory, decided to gaze into its reflective depths after another night of chips and soda.

The Mirror's Reflection

- **Inflammation:** Chronic, low-grade inflammation quietly undermined health, driving metabolic chaos.
- **Anabolic Resistance:** Declining muscle mass made building strength increasingly difficult, accelerating physical decline.

- **Sarcopenia:** Muscle loss led to fat replacement, destabilizing blood sugar, insulin, and cholesterol, leaving the body weak and metabolically dysfunctional.
- **Hormonal Imbalances:** Vital hormones like growth hormone, testosterone, and insulin plummeted, while cortisol surged, wreaking havoc on metabolism and tissue health.
- **Oxidative Stress:** Free radical damage compounded muscle breakdown, delayed recovery, and accelerated aging.

The Result:

Simple acts like standing became monumental challenges, medications piled up, and the joys of movement and connection faded into distant memories. But the mirror also offered hope—a glimpse of what could be with intentional choices:

- A body capable of athleticism, strength, and endurance, no matter the age.

- Freedom to enjoy life, feel fit, and do whatever brings joy, from hiking mountains to dancing at weddings.

- Vitality restored through muscle preservation, balanced hormones, and reduced oxidative stress.

The Pivot Point

Slowly but surely, they began to rewrite their story:

- **Cooking Adventures:** Takeout turned into experiments with vibrant, nutritious meals.
- **Active Downtime:** Netflix marathons became walks or jogs while listening to engaging podcasts.
- **Real Strength Training:** Replacing excuses with actual weights and exercises.
- **Mindful Choices:** Soda was swapped for sparkling water, and chips for a handful of nuts.
- **Rebuilding Bonds:** They reached out to friends and family, rekindling connections over shared meals and laughter.

By the end of their journey, the mirror revealed a different future: vibrant health, joyful relationships, and a legacy of balance and intention. Generation "Now, Not Later" transformed into Generation "Why Not Now?" proving that change is always within reach. So, what chapter are you writing today?

The "YOU" Factor: Discovering the Wealth Within

Imagine a tree rooted in nutrient-rich soil, stretching

its branches skyward to soak in the sun. It doesn't rush to grow taller or twist itself into unnatural shapes to impress the forest—it simply thrives by doing what it was meant to do: absorb, adapt, and flourish. Your body, much like that tree, is designed for resilience, growth, and harmony. But in today's chaotic whirlwind of deadlines, gadgets, and go-go-go culture, we've forgotten how to nurture the soil of our own well-being.

Instead, we treat ourselves like overworked engines running on fumes, patching problems only when the warning lights flash. What if, instead, you could fine-tune your body and mind as a master craftsman refines their tools? What if small, deliberate tweaks could unlock reservoirs of energy, clarity, and joy you didn't know you had?

This book, *Biohacks 101,* is your roadmap to a new way of living. It invites you to approach your well-being with curiosity, experimentation, and intention. By making deliberate, science-backed interventions, you'll uncover reservoirs of energy, clarity, and joy that you may not even know you have.

The Tale of Two Travellers

Let me take you on a mental journey. Picture two travellers embarking on a trek through an endless desert. Both are given the same starting tools and opportunities.

The first traveller, eager to begin, hastily packs whatever is at hand. They grab a bag of random supplies, throw in some water, and set off, reacting to the challenges as they arise. They don't give much thought to pacing, strategy, or resource conservation. The desert soon takes its toll—blistering heat, shifting sands, and thirst lead to exhaustion. Each step feels heavier, each mile more daunting.

The second traveller takes a different approach. Before setting off, they pause to assess their environment. They select lightweight, durable tools and plan their route, incorporating rest stops for recharging. They learn how to navigate sandstorms, ration supplies, and even utilize the environment to their advantage. This traveler moves steadily through the same harsh terrain but with a clear sense of purpose and energy.

Life, for most of us, feels like this desert. The terrain is unforgiving, the demands relentless, and the stakes are high. But here's the truth: you can choose to be the second traveller. Through biohacking—the art of small, intentional improvements—you can thrive in the desert, not just survive it.

A Peek Inside

This book isn't about becoming a superhuman overnight or adding to your to-do list. It's about making life easier, more enjoyable, and sustainable. Here, you'll find practical, science-backed strategies broken into two parts:

Part I: The Foundation of Resilience
- Uncover how an antifragile mindset turns stress into strength.
- Learn to reprogram your subconscious mind, the architect of your habits.
- Cultivate emotional agility and harness the power of relationships to thrive.

Part II: The Hacks That Transform
- Enhance brain function with nourishing foods and mindful nutrition.
- Master techniques like restorative breathing and functional movement for vitality.
- Harness technology and nature-inspired strategies for a healthier, more balanced life.

Let's Begin

Think of this as your blueprint for building a thriving, adaptable life. Each chapter provides a tool to nurture the roots of your health and extend the branches of your potential. Remember: the journey isn't about perfection—it's about progress. You already have the seeds of resilience within you; this guide will show you how to nurture them. Together, we'll explore simple yet powerful ways to transform burnout into brilliance, chaos into clarity, and exhaustion into energy.

2 ANTIFRAGILE MINDSET

"The obstacle is the path." — Zen Proverb.

Antifragility, a concept introduced by Nassim Nicholas Taleb, goes beyond resilience and robustness. While a resilient system withstands adversity and recovers, an antifragile system thrives and grows stronger because of it. It's not about merely enduring challenges but evolving through them.

Nature offers countless metaphors to illustrate this principle. The phoenix rises from ashes, symbolizing renewal and transformation after devastation. Bamboo bends during fierce storms but doesn't break; instead, it stands taller and more resilient. Think of steel, forged in fire, becoming stronger with each strike of the hammer. Or the lotus, blooming magnificently despite the muddy waters surrounding it. Even a diamond—once an unremarkable piece of carbon—achieves brilliance under immense pressure.

These examples remind us that challenges don't define us; our response to them does. The antifragile mindset teaches us to embrace difficulty as an opportunity to grow tougher, smarter, and better.

In our pursuit of growth, it often feels like pushing harder should lead to better outcomes. Yet, sometimes the more we strain, the more elusive success becomes. This is the paradox of the Law of Reversed Effort— true progress often arises from a balance of intention and relaxation, rather than relentless force.

The Stoics, too, emphasized this wisdom: mastering inner resilience and focusing on what we can control. When combined, these principles create a framework for living antifragile—growing stronger through challenges, setbacks, and stressors.

The Art of Kintsugi: A Lesson in Antifragility

The Japanese art of Kintsugi beautifully embodies antifragility. This practice involves repairing broken pottery using lacquer mixed with gold, silver, or platinum. Instead of concealing the cracks, Kintsugi highlights them, creating intricate veins of precious metals. The result? A piece more valuable and beautiful than it was before.

Kintsugi teaches us to see imperfections not as flaws but as marks of resilience and transformation. Like the repaired pottery, we can use life's fractures to become stronger, embracing our history as an integral part of our story.

The Law of Reversed Effort: When Less is More

Sometimes, trying too hard can lead to diminishing returns. The Law of Reversed Effort suggests that by easing up and allowing natural rhythms to guide us, we can unlock our true potential. It's about harnessing the paradoxical power of doing less to achieve more. Here's how to apply this principle in your life:

1. **Balance Focus with Strategic Relaxation**
    *   Action: Alternate between deep focus and intentional pauses.
    *   Why It Works: Neuroscience shows our brains perform best in a state of "relaxed focus," not forced strain.
    *   Practical Example: Plan intense work sprints followed by 5–10 minutes of mindful breathing or movement to reset.

2. **Detach to Recharge**
    *   Action: Step away from problems when feeling stuck.
    *   Why It Works: Breakthroughs often happen

during mental rest, such as walking or engaging in unrelated tasks.

- Practical Example: Use micro-breaks to reset your mind and allow clarity to emerge naturally.

3. **Focus on Process, Not Perfection**
   - Action: Shift your attention from the outcome to the steps you can control.
   - Why It Works: Obsessing over results creates stress, while focusing on the journey sustains motivation.
   - Practical Example: Celebrate small wins and trust the incremental progress

Life's curveballs don't just test us—they shape us. Antifragility is the art of turning challenges into catalysts, setbacks into springboards, and chaos into a canvas for growth. It's not just bouncing back; it's bouncing forward—becoming stronger, wiser, and more adaptable with every twist and turn life throws your way. By weaving small, purposeful actions into the fabric of your daily life, you can cultivate a mindset that doesn't just endure adversity but thrives in it. Let's explore the steps to embrace antifragility and transform pressure into power.

1. **Take Controlled Risks**
   - Action: Step out of your comfort zone daily—whether by trying a new skill, tack-

ling a difficult task, or initiating a bold conversation.

- Why: Controlled risks build confidence, adaptability, and problem-solving abilities.
- Example: Pitch an innovative idea at work or try a new fitness challenge.

2. **Build Your Discomfort Muscle**
   - Action: Incorporate manageable stressors like cold showers, regular exercise, or intermittent fasting.
   - Why: Controlled exposure to discomfort enhances physical and mental resilience over time.
   - Example: Start your day with a 30-second cold shower and gradually increase the duration.

3. **Break Routine with Purpose**
   - Action: Add intentional unpredictability to your day, such as exploring a new route to work, experimenting with a different cuisine, or learning an unconventional skill.
   - Why: Novel experiences stimulate growth, creativity, and adaptability.
   - Example: Join a cultural event or pick up a musical instrument for the first time.

4. **Master Cognitive Reframing**
   - Action: Shift your perspective by viewing

setbacks as opportunities to learn and grow.

- Why: Challenges approached with a positive mindset fuel personal and professional development.
- Example: Reflect on a past failure and identify how it contributed to your current strengths.

5. **Test Small, Fail Small**
   - Action: Run low-stakes experiments, such as pitching an idea, trying a new creative project, or launching a small initiative.
   - Why: Small failures provide invaluable lessons while minimizing risks.
   - Example: Pilot a new business concept with a select group before scaling up.

6. **Build Diverse Connections**
   - Action: Network with people from various cultures, disciplines, and perspectives.
   - Why: Diversity fosters innovation, creativity, and the ability to navigate complex situations.
   - Example: Attend cross-disciplinary meetups or engage with global online communities.

7. **Prioritize Rest and Nutrition**
   - Action: Ensure you get 7–9 hours of quality sleep and eat nutrient-rich, balanced meals.

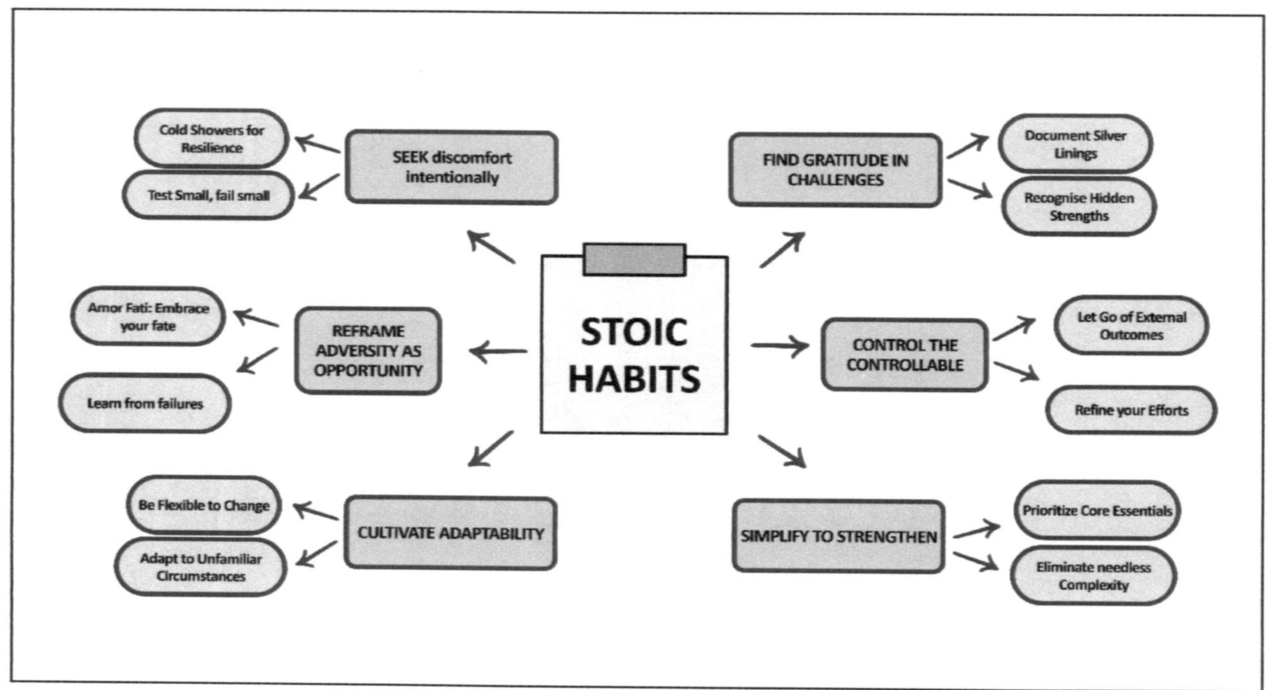

Cold Showers for Resilience
Test Small, fail small
SEEK discomfort intentionally
FIND GRATITUDE IN CHALLENGES
Document Silver Linings
Recognise Hidden Strengths
Amor Fati: Embrace your fate
REFRAME ADVERSITY AS OPPORTUNITY
Learn from failures
STOIC HABITS
CONTROL THE CONTROLLABLE
Let Go of External Outcomes
Refine your Efforts
Be Flexible to Change
CULTIVATE ADAPTABILITY
Adapt to Unfamiliar Circumstances
SIMPLIFY TO STRENGTHEN
Prioritize Core Essentials
Eliminate needless Complexity

- Why: A healthy body is the foundation for a resilient mind.
- Example: Create a consistent evening routine to improve sleep hygiene and prepare brain-fueling meals like those rich in omega-3s and antioxidants.

8. Practice Gratitude and Mindfulness

- Action: Begin each day with journaling, gratitude exercises, or meditation.
- Why: These practices reduce stress, build emotional clarity, and improve resilience.
- Example: Write down three things you're grateful for every morning or spend 10 minutes meditating.

A popular Zen proverb: *"You should sit in meditation for twenty minutes every day—unless you're too busy. Then you should sit for an hour."*

This highlights the importance of mindfulness and self-care, especially during hectic times when it feels counterintuitive to slow down. Busier and more chaotic life becomes, the more essential it is to center yourself through meditation.

9. Adapt and Learn Continuously

- Action: Commit to learning a new skill, hobby, or knowledge area each month.
- Why: Lifelong learning fosters agility in the face of change.

- Example: Take an online course or read a book outside your usual interests.

10. Balance Effort with Rest

- Action: Alternate between focused effort and intentional relaxation, aligning with the Law of Reversed Effort.
- Why: Neuroscience shows that switching between intense work and recovery enhances productivity and creativity.
- Example: Use the Pomodoro technique—work for 25 minutes, then rest for 5 minutes.

By embracing these steps, you cultivate an antifragile mindset that thrives on challenges, learns from adversity, and emerges stronger from every experience.

Three Key Rewards of an Antifragile Life

1. A mind that bounces back.
2. A body primed for health.
3. Relationships that weather storms and flourish.

The Power of Choice

Growth doesn't bloom in comfort—it sparks in those shaky, uncertain moments when you take action despite your fears. The world might whisper, "Wait for the perfect moment," but here's the truth: perfection is a myth. The only thing that matters is starting.

"In the confrontation between the stream and the rock, the stream always wins – not through strength, but by perseverance."
– H. Jackson Brown Jr.

Whether it's opening up a difficult conversation, pitching that daring idea, or taking a bold leap forward, each intentional move nudges you closer to the life you want. Action is the compass that guides you through uncertainty toward possibility.

Closing Thoughts

Strength isn't just about muscles—it's about resilience, grit, and a sense of purpose. Every obstacle you encounter is an invitation to discover new depths of your inner power. Embracing the unknown isn't a gamble—it's a strategy to come out stronger, wiser, and ready for what's next.

Take that first step today. Say yes to action, no to fear. Start small, but start. Build habits that strengthen your resolve, and watch as you rise above challenges and flourish in ways you never imagined.

By blending concepts like the Law of Reversed Effort with Stoic wisdom, you'll learn to navigate pressure, embrace uncertainty, and emerge more resilient from life's trials. Each thought, choice, and action carries the seed of growth. Step boldly. Act with intention. Build an antifragile life—and let adversity become your greatest ally.

3 SUBCONSCIOUS CODE

"The mind is like a radio; tune it wisely, for the frequency you choose determines the life you lead."

—*Roy T. Bennett*

The subconscious mind is the engine of human potential, silently shaping your reality through thoughts, emotions, and beliefs. Like a finely calibrated radio, your mind tunes into specific frequencies—whether high vibrations of love, gratitude, and purpose, or lower ones like fear and doubt—ultimately dictating your experiences. Harnessing the power of your subconscious is not only transformative but essential in achieving emotional well-being, personal growth, and success.

The Science Behind the Subconscious

Mind

1. **Neuroplasticity: Rewiring the Brain**
   - The brain, with its 86 billion neurons, processes up to 70,000 thoughts daily. Remarkably, 95% of these are repetitive, highlighting the subconscious's dominant role.
   - Conscious efforts to replace negative patterns with empowering ones create new neural pathways, fostering resilience and adaptability.

2. **The Role of Brain Waves**
   - Different brain states—Beta (active), Alpha (calm), and Theta (subconscious access)—play distinct roles in rewiring the subconscious.
   - Practices like meditation and visualization help shift from Beta to Alpha and Theta states, enabling deeper transformation.

3. **Hypothalamus: The Control Center**
   - This critical part of the brain governs hormonal balance, emotions, and physical responses.
   - By engaging the subconscious through gratitude and positive affirmation, you influence this control center, fostering calmness and alignment.

Techniques to Harness the Subconscious

1. **Visualization**
   - Action: Picture your desired outcomes with

vivid detail, imagining the emotions, sights, and sounds as if they're real.

- Why it Works: Visualization creates a neurological representation of success, "training" the brain for achievement.

2. Affirmations

- Action: Repeat positive, present-tense statements like "I am capable and calm in all situations."
- Why it Works: Repetition strengthens belief systems, overwriting limiting mental scripts.

3. Gratitude Practices

- Action: Start each day by listing three things you're grateful for.
- Why it Works: Gratitude shifts focus from lack to abundance, activating high-frequency emotions and neural pathways.

4. Meditation

- Action: Dedicate 10–20 minutes daily to focus on your breath, release tension, and connect with elevated emotions.
- Why it Works: Meditation accesses the Alpha and Theta brain states, where subconscious reprogramming is most effective.

5. Sleep Programming

- Action: Feed your mind affirmations or calming thoughts before sleep.
- Why it Works: The subconscious mind stays active during sleep, absorbing and processing inputs received just before and during sleep.
- Affirmations delivered during the transition from alpha to theta states (relaxation to light sleep) are particularly impactful, as the mind becomes highly receptive.
- This programming can influence behavior, emotional resilience, and mental clarity upon waking.

Quantum and Vibrational Biohacks

We are energetic beings, and our vibrations determine our reality. Thoughts, much like the frequency of radio waves, align with specific outcomes. Positive emotions, such as love and enthusiasm, resonate at higher frequencies, attracting opportunities and success, while fear and doubt create interference or 'static'.

Practical Steps to Raise Your Vibration:

1. **Engage in Mindfulness Practices to Cultivate Present-Moment Awareness:**
   - Practice deep breathing: Take 5 minutes daily to focus on slow, deep breaths.
   - Try a mindful activity: Savor a cup of tea, focusing on the aroma, taste, and warmth without distractions.

2. **Surround Yourself with Positive Environments and People:**
   - Declutter your living space to create a calm and inspiring environment.
   - Spend time with friends or mentors who uplift and inspire you.
   - Join a community group, such as a yoga class, book club, or volunteer organization, to connect with
   - like-minded, positive individuals.

3. **Prioritize Actions That Align with Your Values and Goals:**
   - If health is a value, commit to a daily 30-minute workout or prepare nutritious meals.
   - If personal growth is a priority, schedule time to read books or attend workshops in areas of interest.
   - Decline commitments that feel draining or misaligned with your goals, and focus on those that energize you.

Dr. Joe Dispenza's Insights on Neuroplasticity

Dr. Dispenza emphasizes that the mind's power to reshape reality is rooted in neuroplasticity. According to him:

"Nature does not hurry, yet everything is accomplished."
— Lao Tzu

1. **Mind-Body Connection:** The brain doesn't differentiate between real and imagined experiences. Visualizing success can create the same neural patterns as actual achievement.
2. **Elevated Emotions:** Pairing intention with emotions like joy or gratitude forms "new experiences" in the brain, leading to transformation.
3. **Daily Practices:** Commit to meditative practices that integrate intention and emotion, effectively aligning your mind and body.

Imagine you're preparing for a big presentation. If you take time to close your eyes and vividly visualize yourself speaking confidently, engaging the audience, and receiving applause, your brain begins to create the same neural pathways as if you had actually experienced the successful presentation.

This mental rehearsal not only boosts your confidence but also primes your brain to act in alignment with the visualized success when the real moment arrives. Athletes, public speakers, and performers often use this technique to enhance their performance.

Actionable Biohacks for Subconscious Mind Mastery

Subliminal messages are signals or messages designed to bypass the conscious mind and communicate directly with the subconscious. The term "subliminal" means "below the threshold" of conscious perception. The subconscious mind processes vast amounts of information that the conscious mind cannot handle. Subliminal messages aim to tap into this processing power by planting positive or influential ideas directly into the subconscious, potentially creating lasting changes in attitudes or behaviors.

Key Features of Subliminal Messages:

1. **Below Conscious Awareness**:
   Subliminal messages are presented so subtly (e.g., in the form of faint sounds or brief flashes of text) that the conscious mind does not register them, but the subconscious mind does.

2. **Influence on Behavior and Thought Patterns**:
   They aim to influence thoughts, feelings, and behaviors without the individual being actively aware of the influence.

3. **Modes of Delivery**:
   - **Auditory**: Words or affirmations embedded in music or white noise.
   - **Visual**: Quick flashes of text or images in videos, or subtle overlays in graphics.
   - **Kinesthetic**: Subtle tactile inputs, though less common.

Subliminal messages leverage the brain's subconscious processing, tapping into a reservoir of automatic thoughts, beliefs, and biases that operate faster and with more emotional intensity than conscious thought. Neuroscience research, including functional MRI studies, has shown that subliminal stimuli activate brain areas like the limbic system, which governs emotional responses, even without conscious awareness. When repeated, these messages can subtly reinforce specific neural pathways, a process rooted in the brain's neuroplasticity, allowing for habit formation over time. Subliminal messages that incorporate emotionally charged words, such as "love" or "fear," often elicit stronger subconscious reactions, highlighting the power of emotional resonance.

Here are some practical subliminal hacks to subtly train your subconscious mind and make meaningful progress toward your goals:

1. **Use Ambient Background Affirmations**
   - Create a playlist of affirmations aligned with your goals (e.g., confidence, focus, or relaxation).
   - Play it softly in the background while working, relaxing, or sleeping.
     Hack: Keep the volume low enough that it blends with ambient noise but is still perceptible to your subconscious.

2. **Vision Boards with Subliminal Triggers**
   - Design a vision board with images and phrases

that represent your goals.

- Place it somewhere you see daily but don't focus on intensely, like your desk or bedroom wall.

  Hack: Use subtle cues (like color schemes or keywords) that evoke a positive emotional response when glanced at.

3. Subliminal Text Wallpapers

- Use a desktop or phone wallpaper with faint, repeated affirmations embedded in the design.

  Hack: Ensure the text is subtle enough to not distract but still visible enough to register subconsciously.

4. Anchor Positive Messages to Daily Cues

- Pair affirmations with everyday actions, like brushing your teeth or starting your computer.
- For example, stick a post-it note with "I am calm and capable" on your mirror.

  Hack: Change the note regularly to prevent your brain from tuning it out.

5. Gamify Subliminal Training

- Integrate subliminal messages into games or puzzles, like solving crosswords with positive words or playing music with empowering lyrics.

  Hack: Subtle exposure through play helps embed positive associations.

6. **Leverage Peripheral Vision**
   - Place motivational phrases or goal reminders in your peripheral view, such as sticky notes on the edges of your monitor.
   Hack: Your subconscious can register information you don't focus on directly.

7. **Custom Binaural Beats with Affirmations**
   - Pair binaural beats (frequencies designed for relaxation or focus) with affirmations tailored to your goals.
   Hack: Listen while meditating or relaxing to bypass conscious resistance and reinforce messages.

8. **Colour Psychology and Symbols**
   - Surround yourself with colors and symbols associated with your goals (e.g., green for growth, blue for calmness).
   Hack: Use subtle decor changes, like artwork, notebooks, or clothing, to nudge your subconscious.

9. **Subliminal Sticky Note Placement**
   - Write short affirmations on sticky notes and place them in unexpected spots (e.g., inside your cupboard or notebook).
   Hack: Rotating their placement keeps them fresh and surprising for your mind.

10. Create Personalized Mantras in Loops

- Record your voice repeating affirmations and listen while commuting or exercising.
  Hack: Add calming background music to make the experience soothing and enjoyable.

11. Combine with Habit Stacking

- Pair subliminal practices with existing habits, like listening to affirmations while jogging or meditating.
  Hack: Habit stacking reinforces consistency and embeds subliminal exposure effortlessly.

12. Mirror Mantras with Eye Contact

- Write a short affirmation on your mirror and say it out loud while maintaining eye contact.
  Hack: Speaking with conviction reinforces both conscious and subconscious belief.

Why These Hacks Work:

These techniques combine conscious actions with subtle, repeated exposure to positive messages. By engaging multiple senses and integrating them into your routine, they bypass conscious resistance, embedding new beliefs and habits into your subconscious. Here's the table summarizing how to track the effectiveness of subliminal messages on your subconscious mind:

Area of Focus	Tracking Method	Record Outcome
Behavioral Changes	Track specific habits or actions; measure productivity by counting tasks or time spent	After a month of listening to productivity-focused subliminal messages, my weekly task completion increased by 30%.
Mood and Emotional Well-being	Log emotional state daily using a journal or app; rate mood on a scale of 1-10	After three weeks of 20-minute daily listening sessions, my average mood rating improved from 5 to 8.
Cognitive Performance	Challenge focus and memory with tasks like recalling lists or solving puzzles; time yourself recalling details before and after exposure	My memory test score increased by 20% after two weeks of listening to memory-boosting subliminal messages."
Physiological Metrics	Use a smartwatch or device to monitor HRV or sleep patterns; observe changes in resting heart rate	After a month of listening to relaxation subliminal tracks, my heart rate during stressful moments dropped by 5 bpm.

Area of Focus	Tracking Method	Record Outcome
Self-Reported Progress Toward Goals	Reflect weekly on goals and noticeable changes; track weight, meals, and exercise frequency	After two weeks of listening to fitness subliminal messages, I lost 5 pounds and felt more motivated to exercise.
Sleep Quality Improvements	Track sleep duration and quality with apps like Sleep Cycle or Oura Ring; compare deep sleep before and after subliminal practice	After two weeks of listening to subliminal sleep tracks, my deep sleep increased by 20 minutes per night.
Personal Perception of Change	Reflect on personal changes in confidence or focus after daily listening; write journal entries	After a month of confidence-focused subliminal messages, I became more assertive during team meetings.

By applying these tracking methods and reviewing personalized metrics, you can effectively assess the impact of subliminal messages on your subconscious mind and overall well-being.

Closing Thoughts: Tuning Your Inner Radio

The subconscious mind is the bridge between where

you are and where you want to be. By consciously tuning into empowering thoughts and emotions, you can transform every facet of your life. Whether through visualization, meditation, or gratitude, these biohacks rewire your neural pathways, raising your frequency to align with your deepest desires.

Just as a radio emits static until tuned correctly, your life flows effortlessly when aligned with the right mental and emotional frequencies. Master the art of subconscious biohacking, and unlock a limitless mind capable of achieving extraordinary success.

4 URJA: THE BOUNDLESS ENERGY WITHIN

"Everything is energy and that's all there is to it. Match the frequency of the reality you want, and you cannot help but get that reality."

— *Albert Einstein*

Urja, a Sanskrit word for energy, represents the life force flowing through every cell in our body. It's much more than physical vitality—it's a harmony of body, mind, and spirit. Rooted in ancient wisdom and supported by modern science, Urja connects the bioelectric currents within us to our overall well-being. This chapter explores how bioelectricity, meditation, and mindfulness work together to unlock limitless energy, fueling a purposeful and vibrant life.

The Human Body: An Electrical Marvel

Our bodies are living bioelectric systems where energy governs health, movement, and regeneration. Bioelectricity powers key processes like the nervous system, heart rhythms, and cellular functions, extending far beyond the calories we consume.

- **Neurons** transmit electrical signals that control thoughts, movements, and sensations.
- **Heart** relies on rhythmic electrical impulses to sustain circulation.
- **Bones and Skin** exhibit piezoelectric properties, transforming mechanical stress into healing signals.

This intricate web of electrical systems underscores Urja's vital role in maintaining life's vibrancy.

Food Chemistry vs. Bioelectricity

While food provides the raw materials for energy, bioelectricity—produced at the cellular level—is what truly sustains life.

- **Food's Role:** Macronutrients deliver electrons for energy but contribute only 2-3% of the body's vitality.
- **Bioelectricity's Role:** Generated by mitochondrial activity, it accounts for 98% of energy production, supporting cellular communication, healing, and regeneration.

Mitochondria's electron transport chain exemplifies how Urja fuels life beyond physical nourishment.

Bioelectricity and Cellular Programming

Did you know that your cells communicate using tiny electricals and even hold the potential to regenerate lost limbs! Cells exhibit unique electrical identities based on their roles in the body. For instance, nerve cells maintain a resting potential of approximately −70mV, while muscle cells have a resting potential of around −90mV. Diseased or immature cells, such as cancer cells, revert to a neutral electrical state (0 voltage), highlighting the significance of bioelectricity in maintaining cellular identity. Below, we explore the profound implications of bioelectricity in biology.

The Basis of Bioelectric Programming

- Every cell in the human body generates electrical signals through ion channels embedded in its membrane.
- These electrical signals act as instructions that guide cells in their development, function, and interactions with neighboring cells.
- Scientists have discovered that manipulating these bioelectric signals can reprogram cells to adopt specific identities or behaviors. For example: Stem cells can be encouraged to differentiate into specific tissue types.
- Wound Healing: The human body generates electrical currents at injury sites, attracting repair cells and initiating healing processes.

- Cancer Reversal: Cancer cells lose their normal electrical patterns, reverting to a neutral state. By restoring the electrical signature of these cells, experiments have shown that they can be reprogrammed into healthy states, offering a potential breakthrough in cancer therapy.

As research and technology advance, this century may mark a transformative phase in how we understand, manipulate, and leverage the electrical properties of cells to transform our approach to healthcare, offering innovative solutions to some of humanity's most pressing medical challenges.

The connection between energy (Urja) and bioelectricity lies in the fundamental processes that sustain life, where energy is transformed and utilized to generate bioelectric signals. Here's how they are intricately connected:

Urja and bioelectricity are two sides of the same coin, with energy serving as the driving force behind the generation and application of bioelectric signals in biological systems. Understanding their interplay deepens our knowledge of how life functions at both the molecular and holistic levels.

"The cell is the machine, but energy is its lifeblood."
— Dr. Robert O. Becker

Below are some reflections on the connection between the biological and biochemical foundations of bioelectricity, and its ties to traditional healing perspectives."

1. **Energy as the Source of Bioelectricity**
    *   **Cellular Energy Production:** The energy required for generating bioelectricity comes from cellular metabolism, primarily through ATP (adenosine triphosphate) molecules produced in mitochondria. ATP drives ion pumps like the sodium-potassium pump ($Na+/K+$ ATPase), which maintain the electrical potential across cell membranes.
    *   **Urja in the Body:** In ancient texts, "Urja" refers to life-sustaining energy, which can be viewed in modern terms as the biochemical and bioelectric processes powering cells and tissues.

2. **Ion Channels and Electrical Potential**
    *   **Movement of Ions:** Bioelectricity arises from the movement of ions (e.g., sodium, potassium, calcium) across cell membranes. This movement is energy-dependent, relying on ATP to create ion gradients essential for nerve signaling, muscle contraction, and cellular communication.
    *   **Energy's Role:** Without the energy derived from metabolic processes, ion channels and pumps would fail, collapsing the bioelectric

gradients that underlie cellular identity and communication.

3. The Energy Behind Neural Communication and Tissue Healing

- **Nerve Impulses:** The electrical activity in neurons, responsible for transmitting information, is a manifestation of bioelectric energy at work. It converts biochemical energy into bioelectric signals for communication within the body.

- **Healing and Regeneration:** During tissue injury, bioelectric signals guide repair processes. This "healing energy" is driven by the body's ability to redirect metabolic energy into electrical signals that recruit repair cells.

4. Bioelectric Flow

In Holistic and Ancient Healing Systems: Energy (Urja or Prana) is often described as a vital force flowing through the body. Modern bioelectricity parallels this concept:

- **Energy Pathways:** Bioelectric circuits, such as neural networks and cardiac rhythms, align with ideas of energy channels (e.g., nadis in Ayurveda or meridians in Chinese medicine).

- **Electromagnetic Fields:** Bioelectricity creates measurable electromagnetic fields, echoing ancient ideas of a life force surrounding and flowing through the body.

Harnessing Ancient Wisdom and Modern Science

Urja aligns beautifully with ancient concepts like Prana in Vedic traditions and Qi in Chinese medicine, both emphasizing the flow of vital energy.

- **Chakras and Meridians** reflect the nervous system's bioelectric pathways.
- **Meditation and Pranayama** optimize energy flow and coherence.
- **Nature's Energy:** Grounding and sun exposure reconnect us to the Earth's electromagnetic field, enhancing bioelectric potential.

Qi in Martial Arts

Qi is believed to be the inner energy that powers movement, enhances physical strength, and sharpens mental focus. Martial artists train to cultivate, control, and apply Qi effectively. Here's how it relates:

1. **Power Generation (Fa Jin):**
   - Martial artists use Qi to generate explosive power in strikes and movements. This is often linked with proper body alignment, breathing techniques, and mental focus.
   - In styles like Tai Chi or Wing Chun, practitioners talk about harnessing Qi to deliver force efficiently without relying solely on muscle strength.

2. **Breathing Techniques:**
   - Controlled breathing is essential for cultivating Qi. Martial arts forms often synchronize breathing patterns with movements to maximize energy flow.
   - Techniques like Dan Tian breathing focus on the lower abdomen, considered the body's energy center.

3. **Balance and Flow:**
   - Qi is believed to flow through channels in the body called meridians. Maintaining this flow promotes balance, agility, and fluidity in movements.
   - Internal martial arts, like Tai Chi or Bagua Zhang, emphasize the seamless flow of Qi for smooth and effective techniques.

4. **Mental Focus and Awareness:**
   - Qi training enhances a martial artist's ability to remain calm and focused under pressure.
   - This mental clarity is crucial for anticipating an opponent's moves and making precise responses.

5. **Healing and Resilience:**
   - Qi is also associated with health and vitality.
   - Martial arts incorporate Qi-based exercises like

Qigong to build resilience, recover from injuries, and maintain overall well-being.

6. Spiritual Connection:

For many practitioners, cultivating Qi is not just physical but also spiritual. It connects them to the universe and fosters harmony between body, mind, and spirit.

While some aspects of Qi are supported by modern interpretations, like the role of focused breathing and mindfulness, other claims about Qi's metaphysical properties are more philosophical and cultural. Regardless, Qi remains a cornerstone of martial arts traditions, bridging the physical and mental disciplines.

The Transformative Power of Meditation and Mindfulness

Meditation and mindfulness do more than calm the mind; they enhance bioelectric energy flow, promoting balance and resilience.

1. **Brain Function:** Regular meditation boosts alpha and theta brainwave activity, encouraging relaxation, creativity, and clarity.

2. **Heart Rate Variability (HRV):** Improved HRV reflects healthier stress responses and emotional balance.

3. **Stress Reduction:** Mindfulness lowers cortisol levels, boosting overall vitality.

By amplifying neural coherence and physiological efficiency, these practices intensify Urja.

Pranayama: Breath as a Bioelectric Catalyst

Pranayama, or breath control, directly influences bioelectric flow.

- **Improved Oxygenation:** Deep breathing enriches oxygen supply, sharpening mental clarity.
- **Balance:** Alternate nostril breathing harmonizes the brain's hemispheres, fostering calmness.
- **Pineal Gland Activation:** Rhythmic breathing stimulates melatonin production, improving sleep and recovery.

Meditation is a powerful practice that can improve mental clarity, emotional stability, and physical health. To get the most out of it, here are some detailed guidelines:

1. Set the Right Environment

Creating the right atmosphere helps deepen your meditation practice:

- Quiet Space: Find a calm, quiet place where you won't be disturbed.
- Lighting: Use soft lighting or candles to create a serene ambiance.

- Comfortable Seat: Sit on a cushion, chair, or mat to maintain an upright posture without strain.
- Aroma: Use essential oils or incense (e.g., lavender, sandalwood) to relax your senses.
- Minimal Distractions: Turn off devices or put them on silent mode.

2. Establish a Daily Routine

- Timing: Meditate at the same time each day (e.g., early morning or evening).
- Duration: Start with 5–10 minutes and gradually increase to 20–30 minutes.
- Consistency: Practice daily for cumulative benefits.

3. Posture and Breathing

Posture:

- Sit upright with a straight spine. Relax your shoulders.
- Rest your hands on your knees or in your lap.

Breathing:

- Breathe deeply through the nose, expanding your diaphragm.
- Use rhythmic or box breathing (e.g., inhale for 4 seconds, hold for 4, exhale for 4, hold for 4).

4. Visualization Techniques

Visualizations enhance focus and align your intentions:

Light Visualization:

- Imagine a warm, golden light entering through the crown of your head and filling your body with peace.
- Picture this light cleansing negative energy and illuminating your bioelectric pathways.

Nature Imagery:

- Visualize yourself in a serene place, like a forest, beach, or mountain.
- Imagine feeling connected to the Earth's energy.

Energy Flow:

- Visualize energy moving along your body's meridians or chakras.
- See it as a glowing current revitalizing your body.

Goals and Healing:

Imagine achieving a personal goal or healing a part of your body with your mind's energy.

Harnessing Bioelectric Harmony for Mind and Body

1. Ever wondered how to stay composed in emotional moments?
2. Are you searching for deeper meaning in life?
3. What if you could sharpen your mind in just 10 minutes a day, enhancing your focus and productivity?
4. Are you feeling overwhelmed by life's pressures?

5. Struggling to fall asleep at night?

6. Did you know that peace of mind can boost your overall health?

7. What if your mind could become a fertile ground for creativity?

Who doesn't love simplicity?

Meditation provides the answers to these questions, and the best part is that it's accessible and easy to start. It's a simple habit that offers profound benefits, helping you grow stronger, healthier, and more connected to your true self.

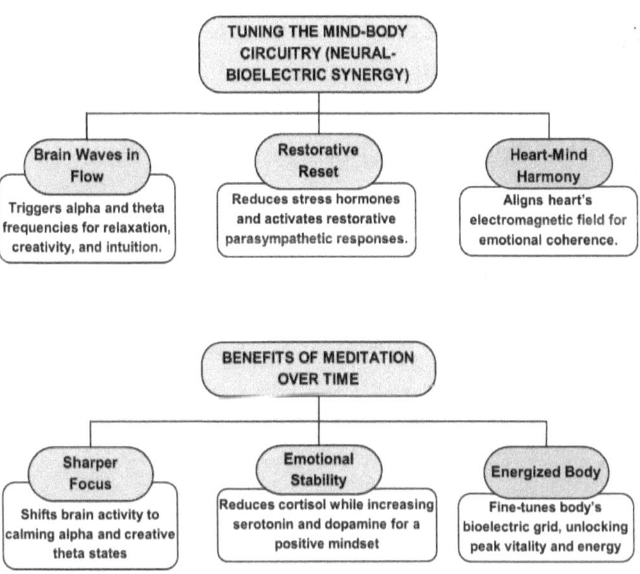

Closing Thoughts

With great power comes great responsibility, and achieving more requires a steady mind and a resilient body. Meditation is the key to this harmony—a practice that aligns the body's bioelectric rhythms, balances neural activity, and fosters inner peace. By calming the mind through alpha and theta brainwave states and activating the parasympathetic nervous system, meditation eases stress and enhances creativity. Its ability to bridge the heart and mind through electromagnetic coherence unlocks an endless loop of vitality, focus, and resilience. Now is the time to adapt—make meditation a daily ritual to not only sustain your energy but to amplify it, fueling your aspirations while maintaining emotional and physical well-being.

5 BOX BREATHING

"Almost everything will work again if you unplug it. Including you."

—Anne Lamott

Box breathing, also known as square breathing, is a powerful and accessible biohacking technique that has been adopted by everyone from elite Navy SEALs to mindfulness practitioners. It involves a rhythmic breathing pattern that can help you reduce stress, sharpen your focus, and enhance your overall well-being. Here's how it works and why it's a game-changer for biohackers like you.

What is Box Breathing?

Box breathing is a controlled breathing exercise that follows a specific pattern: inhale, hold, exhale, hold, each for the same amount of time. This simple yet profound technique activates the body's natural relaxation response, helping you regain control over your nervous system and bring balance to your mind and body.

It's called "box breathing" because each phase of the breath (inhale, hold, exhale, hold) is the same length, creating a balanced "box" in your breath cycle. It's easy to learn, adaptable to any setting, and most importantly, effective.

How to Perform Box Breathing

The beauty of box breathing lies in its simplicity. Here's how you can practice it:

- **Inhale:** Slowly breathe in through your nose for 4 seconds, filling your lungs with air.
- **Hold:** Hold your breath for 4 seconds. Focus on the stillness during this pause.
- **Exhale:** Gently breathe out through your mouth for 4 seconds, releasing all the air.
- **Pause:** Hold your breath again for 4 seconds before starting the next cycle.

Repeat this cycle 4–5 times, or as needed. As you get comfortable, feel free to adjust the timing to suit your preference—some biohackers even extend each phase to 6 or 8 seconds for deeper relaxation.

The Origins of Box Breathing

Though the technique has gained widespread popularity in the wellness and mindfulness communities, Box

Breathing originally emerged as a method for Navy SEALs and other special combat units to manage stress and maintain composure under extreme pressure. The ability to stay calm and focused in high-stress situations can make the difference between success and failure, and box breathing was developed as a practical tool to achieve that balance.

Today, box breathing has evolved beyond the military and is a go-to strategy for anyone looking to enhance focus, calm the mind, and manage stress—whether you're preparing for a big presentation, dealing with anxiety, or simply seeking a moment of peace in a busy day.

The Neuroscience of Box Breathing

When we're stressed, the body activates the sympathetic nervous system, triggering the "fight-or-flight" response. This causes an increase in heart rate, faster breathing, and elevated levels of cortisol—the stress hormone. Over time, chronic stress can wreak havoc on both the mind and body, leading to issues like anxiety, depression, and high blood pressure.

Box breathing works by stimulating the parasympathetic nervous system, also known as the "rest-and-digest" system. This activation triggers a state of relaxation, slowing the heart rate and lowering blood pressure. Regular practice has been shown to reduce cortisol levels, improve emotional regulation, and restore balance to the nervous system.

By slowing down and consciously controlling your breath, you're not only calming your body, but you're also enhancing your ability to focus, think clearly, and act with intention.

The Benefits of Box Breathing

The power of box breathing goes far beyond simply calming the mind. When practiced regularly, it can provide a multitude of benefits:

- **Stress and Anxiety Reduction:** Box breathing is an excellent tool for reducing stress, managing anxiety, and cultivating a sense of calm in even the most chaotic of situations.
- **Mental Clarity:** By improving oxygenation to the brain, it enhances focus, concentration, and cognitive function. It's especially useful when you need to sharpen your mind before a big decision, exam, or creative task.
- **Improved Sleep:** Box breathing before bedtime can significantly enhance your sleep quality, helping you fall asleep faster and achieve deeper, restorative rest.
- **Enhanced Emotional Regulation:** By calming the nervous system, box breathing helps reduce emotional reactivity, making it easier to

maintain composure during stressful encounters.

- **Stronger Immune System:** Consistent practice helps lower cortisol levels, which in turn boosts the immune system, making you more resilient to illness.
- **Increased Performance:** Whether you're an athlete or just facing a high-pressure moment at work, box breathing can enhance your physical performance by improving endurance, focus, and recovery.

Integrating Box Breathing into Daily Life

The beauty of box breathing is that it can be practiced anywhere, at any time. You don't need a yoga mat or a quiet space—just a few minutes of your day to reset your system. Here are some ways to incorporate it into your routine:

- **Before Big Meetings or Presentations:** Use box breathing to calm your nerves and enhance your focus before stepping into a high-pressure situation.
- **In Between Tasks:** When juggling multiple projects, take a moment to perform a few cycles of box breathing to regain clarity and energy.

"Worry often gives a small thing a big shadow."

– Swedish Proverb

- **During Exercise:** Box breathing can be used to calm your mind during workouts, aiding in endurance and recovery.
- **When Feeling Overwhelmed:** Box breathing can serve as a quick reset when life feels chaotic—just take a moment to breathe deeply and re-center.
- **Pre-Bedtime Ritual:** Incorporate box breathing into your evening routine to quiet your mind and prepare your body for restful sleep.

Customizing Your Box Breathing Practice

While the classic 4-4-4-4 pattern is a great starting point, don't be afraid to personalize the practice based on your needs. Some people find that extending the inhale and exhale to 5 or 6 seconds helps them relax even more deeply, while others may benefit from a shorter cycle. Here are a few variations to try:

- 4-4-6-2: A longer exhale and shorter pause for deeper relaxation.
- 6-2-6-2: A more extended cycle to enhance focus and mental clarity.
- 3-3-3-3: A quicker cycle for a fast reset when you need it most.

Closing Thoughts: The Science of Consistency

Like any biohacking practice, the true benefits of box breathing emerge through measurable consistency.

Studies suggest that practicing box breathing for just 5 minutes daily over a period of 8 weeks can significantly lower cortisol levels by up to 25%, enhance heart rate variability (HRV) by 15%, and reduce symptoms of anxiety by 30%. By making box breathing a routine habit, you train your nervous system to handle stress with increased resilience and control. With time and persistence, this technique becomes a powerful tool for staying calm, focused, and in charge, even in the face of life's challenges.

Whether you aim to reduce stress, boost performance, or improve sleep quality, this scientifically-supported practice delivers. Commit to just 5-10 minutes daily, follow the rhythm of the box, and witness how this simple yet effective habit transforms your mind, body, and overall well-being.

6 THE EMOTIONAL EDGE

"Your emotions are the slaves to your thoughts,
and you are the slave to your emotions."

— *Elizabeth Gilbert*

Emotional wellbeing transcends the idea of merely managing emotions—it's about mastering them to optimize mental health, strengthen relationships, and make better decisions. Emotional Intelligence (EI) is a powerful mental biohack that empowers individuals to turn emotions into tools for productivity, resilience, and happiness.

The Pillars of Emotional Intelligence

1. Self-Awareness
- Action: Identify and understand your emotions as they arise.
- Why It Matters: Being self-aware allows for

better stress regulation and decision-making.

2. Self-Regulation
- Action: Control impulses and manage reactions thoughtfully.
- Why It Matters: Enables you to respond thoughtfully rather than react emotionally in challenging situations.

3. Empathy
- Action: Tune into and understand the feelings of others.
- Why It Matters: Builds trust, reduces conflict, and fosters stronger relationships.

4. Social Skills
- Action: Cultivate adaptability, active listening, and clear communication.
- Why It Matters: Effective social skills are essential for success in both personal and professional contexts.

5. Motivation
- Action: Align your goals with a deeper sense of purpose to sustain long-term drive.
- Why It Matters: Helps navigate adversity while staying focused on meaningful objectives.

The Science of Emotional Wellbeing

Emotions are deeply rooted in neurobiology, involving a complex interplay between different brain regions and hormones.

- **Amygdala vs. Prefrontal Cortex:** Emotional intelligence helps shift control from the reactive amygdala (fear center) to the rational prefrontal cortex, enabling thoughtful decision-making.
- **Neurochemical Drivers:** Mirror neurons foster empathy by allowing us to feel others' emotions, while oxytocin strengthens trust and collaboration.
- **Rewiring the Brain:** Practices like gratitude and mindfulness can reshape neural pathways, fostering resilience and long-term emotional stability.

Practical Steps to Cultivate Emotional Intelligence

1. **Show Empathy**
   - Empathy is about understanding, not fixing.
   - Neuroscience Insight: Mirror neurons help us experience others' emotions, deepening trust and reducing conflict.

2. **Pause Before Reacting**
   - Emotional outbursts are triggered by the amygdala. A simple pause activates the prefrontal cortex, enabling reasoned responses.

- Action: Take a deep breath or count to three before responding in emotionally charged situations.

3. Assume Good Intent
- The brain naturally perceives threats faster than rewards. Shifting your mindset to assume positive intent fosters collaboration.
- Action: Ask questions and seek clarification instead of jumping to conclusions.

4. Practice Gratitude
- Gratitude rewires the brain for positivity and reduces stress.
- Action: Start or end your day by writing down three things you're grateful for.

5. Own Your Mistakes
- Vulnerability builds trust. Admitting faults fosters growth and credibility.
- Action: Replace defensiveness with accountability.

6. Lift Others Up
- Acts of encouragement release dopamine for both the giver and the receiver, creating an atmosphere of positivity.
- Action: Celebrate the successes of others, offer mentorship, and express genuine appreciation.

7. Build Reliable Relationships

- Trust is built on keeping promises, which releases oxytocin and strengthens bonds.
- Action: Follow through on commitments consistently.

Managing Anger: The Hormone Hijacker

Anger is a natural response, but when left unchecked, it becomes a health hazard. It hijacks your hormonal balance, flooding the body with adrenaline and cortisol—the stress hormones. These not only strain your heart and mind but also impair decision-making and relationships. As Ambrose Bierce wisely said, *"Speak when you are angry, and you will make the best speech you will ever regret."* Learning to pause, breathe, and channel anger constructively can transform it from a destructive force into a catalyst for growth and understanding.

Short-Term Impacts

- Elevated heart rate and blood pressure strain the cardiovascular system.
- Suppressed immune function makes you more susceptible to illness.
- Muscle tension and headaches.
- Impaired judgment and cognitive clarity.

Long-Term Impacts

- Chronic stress increases the risk of anxiety and

depression.

- Damaged relationships due to unresolved conflicts.
- Detrimental effects on physical health, including heart disease and digestive issues.

Quick Biohacks to Manage Anger

- **Deep Breathing:** Inhale deeply through your nose, hold, and exhale slowly.
- **Meditation**: A few minutes of meditation can significantly reduce reactivity.
- **Physical Activity:** Exercise is a powerful outlet for releasing pent-up energy.
- **Nature Therapy:** Spending time outdoors reduces stress and promotes calmness.

Emotional Alchemy: Turning Feelings into Fuel

Transforming emotions like stress and anger into motivation and growth is the hallmark of emotional mastery. The following practices can help:

- **Journaling:** Reflect on challenging experiences and reframe them as lessons.
- **Visualization:** Imagine the person you aspire to become and align your actions with that vision.
- **Connection:** Strengthen relationships by fostering trust, expressing gratitude, and practicing empathy.

"You will not be
punished for your
anger; you will be
punished by your
anger."
– Buddha

RECLAIM EMOTIONS

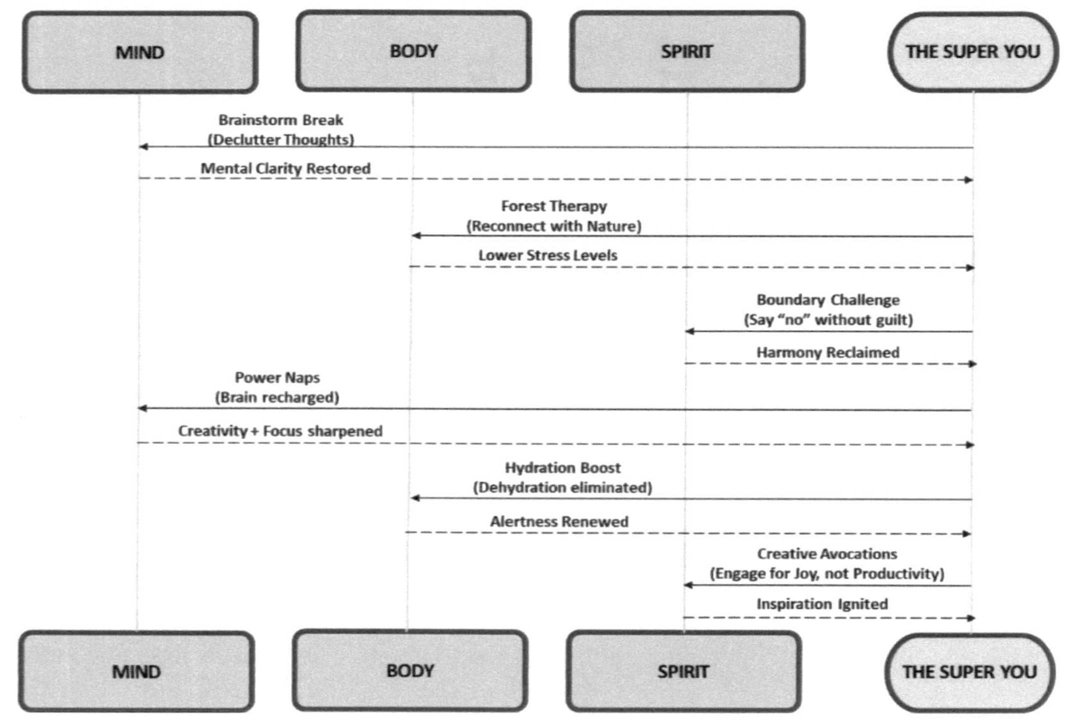

Still as a Mountain, Steady as the Tide

Emotional balance is like standing firm on solid ground, unaffected by the winds of chaos. It begins with self-awareness, the cornerstone of inner peace. By understanding the roots of our emotions and the triggers that sway them, we can choose to respond with intention rather than reacting on impulse. A deep breath, a moment of reflection, or a mindful shift in focus can serve as the gentle anchor that keeps us steady.

Our bodies, too, are integral to emotional regulation. Gentle stretches to release tension, staying hydrated to nourish the mind, or stepping outdoors to embrace nature's calming rhythm all help reset the system. Rituals like journaling or immersing in soothing melodies transform overwhelming emotions into a tapestry of clarity and calm.

On a deeper level, emotional resilience flourishes when we reconnect with what truly matters. By nurturing gratitude, setting healthy boundaries, and realigning with personal values, we reclaim our energy and purpose. When actions harmonize with aspirations, we cultivate a life rooted in balance, creating an unshakable foundation for the soul.

Closing Thoughts

Emotions are powerful signals, guiding our decisions, shaping our connections, and reflecting our inner state.

By cultivating emotional awareness, we shift from being reactive to responsive, reclaiming control over how we navigate life's highs and lows. This process involves recognizing emotions without judgment, decoding their messages, and channeling their energy toward purposeful action. In reclaiming emotion, we transcend mere survival to thrive with authenticity, resilience, and a deeper sense of self-mastery.

7 SOCIAL NETWORK

"Connection is why we're here; it gives purpose and meaning to our lives."

— *Brené Brown*

Humans are inherently wired for connection. Every interaction, gesture, and conversation shapes not only our well-being but also our identity. A robust social network serves as the cornerstone of a fulfilling life, while understanding the dynamics of connection enables us to thrive in an increasingly complex world.

Neuroscience reveals that social bonding is more than an emotional experience—it's a physiological process rooted in hormones, neural pathways, and the brain's reward systems. Let's explore the architecture of human connection and practical ways to enhance our social and mental resilience.

The Architecture of Connection

Our brains are biologically designed to decode subtle social cues such as tone of voice, body language, and micro-expressions.

- **How It Works**:
  What we often call "intuition" is the brain rapidly processing intricate patterns to predict intentions and outcomes.
- **Why It Matters:**
  Understanding these cues helps build meaningful relationships, foster collaboration, and navigate social dynamics effectively.

The Pain of Exclusion

Social rejection impacts us deeply—not just emotionally but neurologically. It registers in the brain in a manner similar to physical pain, underscoring the critical role of inclusion and belonging in mental health.

- **Impact on Well-Being:**
  Repeated rejection can lead to chronic stress, anxiety, and a diminished sense of self-worth.
- **What You Can Do:**
  Seek environments that prioritize inclusivity and cultivate a network where you feel valued and respected.

Relationships Rewire the Brain

Long-term relationships—be they friendships, family

bonds, or romantic connections—reshape neural pathways tied to stress regulation, emotional stability, and cognitive function.

- **Science Says:**
Positive relationships increase oxytocin, the "bonding hormone," which reduces cortisol, the stress hormone.
- **Key Takeaway:**
It's not just about how many connections you have but the quality and nurturance of those relationships that matter most.

The Science of Influence

Why do some people naturally inspire trust while others struggle to connect? Social neuroscience shows that our brains instinctively respond to authenticity, empathy, and perceived competence.

- **Leveraging Influence:**
Align actions with values, demonstrate authenticity, and practice active listening to build trust.
- **Practical Application:**
Clear communication and empathy enhance your ability to influence others positively and inspire collaboration.

"Build your
network before you
need it"
– Tanya Hal

People Radar: Mastering the Art of Understanding and Dealing with Others

The World is a Mixed Bag. In every corner of life, you'll encounter people who uplift you and others who challenge your boundaries. The key to thriving in this world is not to avoid these encounters but to build the emotional and cognitive skills necessary to assess and interact with different types of personalities.

1. Sharpen Your People-Reading Skills

- Observe Body Language: Learn to interpret non-verbal cues like eye contact, posture, and micro-expressions.
- Listen Actively: Focus on both what is being said and what is left unsaid. Pay attention to silences and pauses, as they often carry significant meaning.
- Gauge Intentions: Ask yourself, "What motivates this person?" Understanding someone's goals often reveals their character.

2. Develop a Balanced Perspective

- Recognize the Spectrum: No one is purely good or bad. People's actions are often shaped by circumstances, insecurities, or unmet needs.
- Avoid Overgeneralizing: Assess behavior in context rather than labeling someone based on a single action.

3. Build Emotional Resilience

- Detach from Negativity: Practice boundaries to protect yourself from draining or toxic interactions.
- Cultivate Empathy: Understanding why someone behaves poorly doesn't excuse it but can help you respond wisely.
- Stay Grounded: Use mindfulness techniques to manage your emotions and avoid being reactive.

4. Master the Art of Interaction

- Dealing with Good People: Celebrate their strengths, build trust, and nurture healthy relationships.
- Navigating Challenging Individuals: Be firm yet fair. Establish clear boundaries and communicate assertively without aggression.

5. Learn and Adapt

Every interaction, whether positive or negative, is an opportunity to refine your skills. Treat people as teachers: learn what to emulate and what to avoid.

6. Cultivate Your Inner Compass

- Trust Your Intuition: Your gut often senses red flags or green lights before your mind does.
- Align with Values: Surround yourself with individuals who inspire and reflect your core

principles.

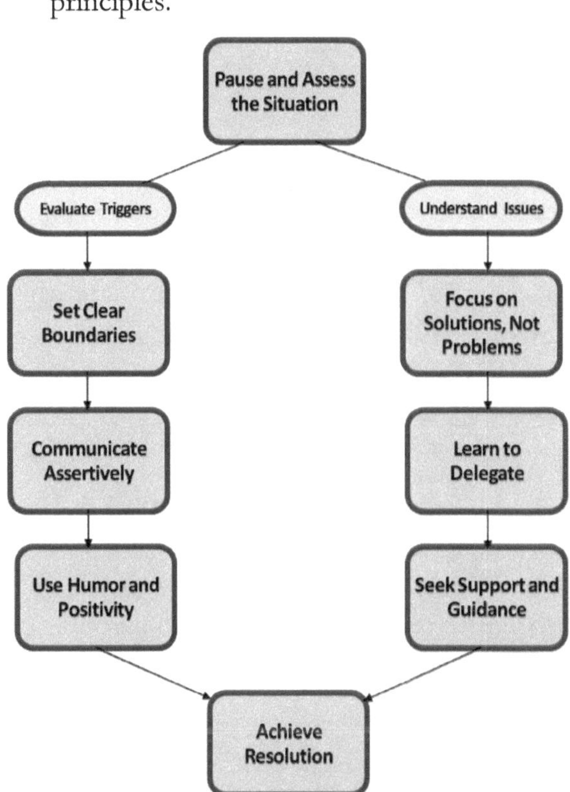

Closing Thoughts: Connection as a Practice

Mastering the art of assessing and dealing with people is a lifelong skill that pays dividends in both personal and professional life. By honing your awareness, emotional intelligence, and adaptability, you can navigate the complexities of human interactions with confidence and wisdom.

Remember: the world is a mosaic of personalities. Your

task isn't to sort the good from the bad but to recognize each piece for what it is—and decide how it fits into your own life.

Your social network is not just a collection of acquaintances—it is a dynamic support system shaping your mental, physical, and emotional well-being. By nurturing meaningful relationships, balancing empathy with boundaries, and fostering habits like gratitude, mindfulness, and reflection, you can create a resilient and thriving social ecosystem.

Every interaction offers an opportunity to grow stronger and more connected. By mastering the art of human connection, you not only strengthen your network but also transform your life with purpose and joy.

8 NUTRITIONAL WISDOM

"Fuel your body like it's worth a million dollars - because it is."

— Dr. Mark Hyman

The Trap of Extreme Practices

Why chase the stars when the earth offers its abundance? In our relentless quest for health and longevity, we are often seduced by the dazzling promise of extremes—implants designed to replace our body's natural functions, gene editing that tinkers with our DNA, plasma exchange touted as the fountain of youth, miracle drugs promising instant results, and futuristic elixirs that claim to defy aging itself. These innovations, while remarkable, often distract us from the most potent and accessible tools for vitality.

The secret to a healthy life doesn't always require

breakthroughs from a laboratory or interventions borrowed from science fiction. It lies in the fundamental principles of nature—principles that have sustained humanity for millennia. The soil beneath our feet nurtures vibrant, life-giving foods. The rhythms of the earth provide balance and harmony. The wisdom of nature teaches us how to flourish, if only we pause to listen.

This chapter is an invitation to step back from the brink of extremes and embrace the profound simplicity of nourishment as nature intended. By reconnecting with the basics—whole foods, mindful movement, restorative rest, and meaningful connections—we rediscover the sustainable path to true health.

No One-Size-Fits-All Approach

When it comes to nutrition, one truth stands tall: there's no universal diet that works for everyone. Our unique genetics, lifestyles, and cultural influences make personalized eating a cornerstone of health. Instead of chasing the latest fads, it's wiser to embrace a flexible and mindful approach that suits your body's needs.

Eating Mindfully, Eating Intuitively

Modern life often disconnects us from the act of eating. Mindful eating—being fully present during meals—can bridge this gap. It involves paying attention to hunger cues, savoring flavors, and honoring satiety.

- Actionable Tip: Pause before each meal to assess your hunger level. Eat slowly, chew thoroughly, and listen to your body's signals.
- **Why It Matters:** Mindful eating reduces overeating, improves digestion, and fosters a healthier relationship with food.

Family and Cultural Roots in Nutrition

Food traditions often hold centuries of wisdom. Recipes passed down through generations are typically rich in seasonal, locally available, and nutritionally dense ingredients.

- **Takeaway:** Honor your family's eating patterns but balance them with modern science.
- **Example:** If your family enjoys carb-rich meals, pair them with fiber-rich vegetables to manage blood sugar spikes.

Eat Foods in the Right Order

Jessie Inchauspé, a French biochemist, also known as the "Glucose Goddess," offers a simple yet transformative strategy for managing blood sugar: eat foods in a specific order during meals. By prioritizing the sequence of vegetables, proteins, fats, and carbohydrates, you can significantly reduce glucose spikes and their after effects.

1. **Start with Vegetables or Fiber**
   Kick off your meal with non-starchy vegetables or fiber-rich foods. These create a "fiber mesh" in your gut, slowing digestion and reducing glucose absorption.
   - Why: Fiber acts as a protective barrier, moderating the release of sugar into your bloodstream.
   - Examples: Leafy greens, broccoli, zucchini, or a fresh salad.

2. **Add Proteins and Fats**
   Next, include proteins and healthy fats. These further decelerate digestion and help stabilize your blood sugar levels.
   - Why: Proteins and fats blunt the glycemic impact of the carbohydrates you'll eat later.
   - Examples: Chicken, fish, eggs, cheese, avocado, or a handful of nuts.

3. **Finish with Carbohydrates**
   Save starchy or sugary foods for last. By consuming them after fiber, protein, and fat, their effect on your blood sugar is significantly diminished.
   - Why: The earlier foods act like a shield, minimizing sharp glucose spikes and crashes.
   - Examples: Rice, pasta, bread, or a small dessert.

Why This Order Works
   - Starting with fiber slows glucose absorption by

creating a protective gel in your gut.

- Following with proteins and fats steadies the release of sugar into your bloodstream.
- Eating carbohydrates last minimizes blood sugar spikes, keeping energy levels consistent and reducing cravings.

Practical Tip

If you can't control the order perfectly—like during a family meal or dining out—try having a fiber-rich starter, such as a small salad or some steamed greens, before indulging in carb-heavy dishes.

The Vicious Sugar Cycle: A Hidden Enemy

The cycle begins deceptively: a sugary meal triggers a surge of glucose in your bloodstream. Your body responds by flooding your system with insulin to bring blood sugar levels back down. This rapid drop leaves you feeling drained and craving more sugar for an instant energy boost. You give in, setting off another wave of glucose and insulin, creating a relentless cycle.

How Glucose Spikes Affect Long-Term Health

1. **Increased Risk of Type 2 Diabetes:**
   Repeated glucose spikes lead to insulin resistance, where cells become less responsive to insulin. This is a precursor to type 2 diabetes.
2. **Chronic Inflammation:**

High glucose levels trigger inflammation, which is associated with heart disease, obesity, and other chronic conditions.

3. **Hormonal Imbalances:**
Conditions like PCOS (Polycystic Ovary Syndrome) and menopause-related symptoms can worsen due to fluctuating glucose levels.

4. **Cardiovascular Issues:**
Glucose spikes contribute to arterial damage, increasing the risk of hypertension, atherosclerosis, and heart attacks.

5. **Accelerated Aging:**
Elevated glucose levels over time lead to glycation,

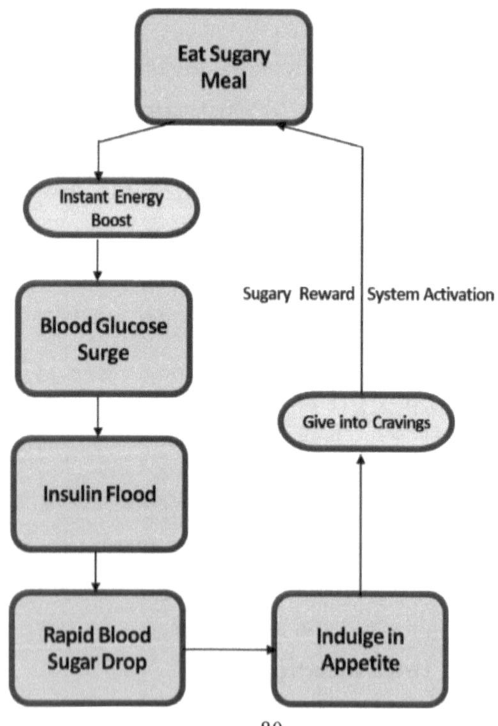

where sugars attach to proteins and DNA, damaging cells and promoting aging.

6. **Mental Health and Energy:**
Chronic spikes affect mood stability and cognitive function due to fluctuating energy levels.

Breaking free from this trap isn't simply about eliminating sugar altogether. It's about reclaiming balance and restoring your body's natural ability to regulate blood sugar before the cycle spirals further out of control.

The Glucose Goddess Mantra

- **Stop Counting Calories:** Calories don't reveal how food impacts glucose levels. Focus on the quality of food rather than quantity.
- **Prioritize Savory Breakfasts:** Avoid sugary breakfasts to maintain energy levels and prevent cravings throughout the day.
- **Dress Your Carbs:** Add protein, fiber, or fats to your carbs to reduce their glucose impact.
- **75% Reduction:** Starting meals with vegetables can cut glucose spikes by 75%, highlighting the profound impact of order of food intake on long term health.
- **30% Reduction:** Drinking a tablespoon of vinegar diluted in water before a meal reduces glucose spikes by 30%.

- **Minutes Movement:** A simple post-meal activity lasting 10 minutes can significantly improve glucose management.

Global Wisdom: Key Nutritional Insights from Around the World

1. **Dr. Jonny Bowden's Global Guide to Vibrant Nutrition**
   - **Power Up with Nutrient-Dense Plates:** Enjoy a rainbow of foods like Japan's sushi bowls, India's lentil dal, or Mexico's guacamole with fresh veggies.
   - **Low-Carb, High-Fat Fusion:** Savor Mediterranean olive-topped salads, buttery ghee-infused Indian curries, or grilled avocado and salmon tacos.
   - **Inflammation Fighters on the Go:** Sip golden turmeric lattes in Asia or indulge in ginger-spiced soups in Europe to keep inflammation at bay.
   - **Balanced Blood Sugar, Anytime:** Kickstart your day with protein-rich tamagoyaki (Japanese omelet) or an avocado toast spin in California style.
   - **Superfoods from Every Corner:** Relish matcha tea in Kyoto, açai bowls in Brazil, or the crunch of kimchi in South Korea for a nutrient boost.
   - **Mindful Morsels:**

Make meals an experience—whether you're savoring sushi rolls in Japan or street pho in Vietnam, pause and enjoy.

- **Personalized Plates:**
Blend global flavors, like pairing Asian stir-fries with low-GI quinoa, to suit your unique palate and health goals.

2. Dr. Michael Greger – Nutrition and Longevity

Dr. Greger champions plant-based eating to prevent chronic diseases and enhance longevity. His book *How Not to Die* underscores the power of whole, unprocessed foods like fruits, vegetables, legumes, and nuts. The Daily Dozen Checklist by Dr. Greger is a powerful tool for promoting optimal health through a plant-based, nutrient-dense diet. It emphasizes a balanced approach to eating that includes a wide variety of foods to ensure you get all the essential nutrients your body needs to thrive. Here's why it's important:

- **Nutrient Diversity**
The checklist encourages eating a variety of foods—beans, fruits, vegetables, nuts, seeds, whole grains, and spices—ensuring that your body receives a broad spectrum of vitamins, minerals, and antioxidants. This diversity supports all bodily systems, from immune function to cognitive health.

"The state of your gut determines the state of your mind."

– Dr. Natasha Campbell-McBride

- **Supports Weight Management**
Many of the items on the Daily Dozen are high in fiber and low in calories, which can help with satiety and regulate blood sugar levels. This combination makes it easier to maintain a healthy weight.
- **Reduces Chronic Disease Risk**
Dr. Greger's checklist includes foods that are rich in antioxidants and anti-inflammatory compounds, which may lower the risk of chronic diseases such as heart disease, cancer, and diabetes. For example, cruciferous vegetables and berries are linked to cancer prevention, while whole grains and beans help lower cholesterol and regulate blood sugar.
- **Promotes Gut Health**
Many of the foods recommended (such as beans, flaxseeds, and vegetables) are rich in fiber, which supports a healthy gut microbiome. A well-balanced microbiome is crucial for digestion, immune health, and even mental well-being.
- **Improves Energy and Mental Clarity**
By focusing on whole, plant-based foods and minimizing processed foods, the Daily Dozen can help optimize your metabolism and provide steady, long-lasting energy. Nutrient-dense foods also support brain health, potentially improving focus and cognitive function.
- **Sustainability and Prevention**

The Daily Dozen emphasizes plant-based foods that are not only good for your health but also have a lower environmental impact compared to animal products. By eating more plants and fewer animal-based foods, you contribute to a more sustainable food system.

- **Easy-to-Follow Framework**
The checklist is simple and easy to integrate into daily life. By just aiming to include a variety of foods each day, you can confidently ensure that you're covering all your nutritional bases without the stress of complex meal planning.

Here's how you can organize Dr. Greger's Daily Dozen Checklist into meal and workout sections:

Morning:
1. **Beans** (½ cup cooked lentils or chickpeas)
2. **Berries** (½ cup blueberries or raspberries)
3. **Greens** (1 cup raw spinach or kale)
4. **Whole Grains** (½ cup cooked oats or quinoa)
5. **Beverages** (1 cup water or herbal tea)
6. **Flaxseeds** (1 tablespoon ground flaxseed added to smoothie or oatmeal)
7. **Nuts and Seeds** (¼ cup walnuts or 2 tablespoons almond butter)

Mid-Morning Snack:
1. **Other Fruits** (1 medium apple or banana)

2. **Spices** (A pinch of cinnamon or turmeric in your tea or smoothie)
3. **Beverages** (1 cup water or green tea)

Lunch:
1. **Cruciferous Vegetables** (½ cup cooked broccoli or Brussels sprouts)
2. **Other Vegetables** (1 cup raw bell peppers or carrots)
3. **Beans** (½ cup cooked black beans or split peas)
4. **Whole Grains** (½ cup cooked brown rice or whole wheat bread)
5. **Beverages** (1 cup water or herbal tea)

Mid-Afternoon Snack:
1. **Other Fruits** (1 medium orange or mango)
2. **Nuts and Seeds** (¼ cup sunflower seeds or 2 tablespoons peanut butter)
3. **Beverages** (1 cup green tea)

Dinner:
1. **Greens** (½ cup cooked Swiss chard or mustard greens)
2. **Cruciferous Vegetables** (1 cup raw kale or cauliflower)
3. **Beans** (½ cup cooked chickpeas or lentils)
4. **Whole Grains** (½ cup cooked quinoa or whole wheat bread)
5. **Beverages** (1 cup water)

Exercise Session:

Goal: 90 minutes of moderate activity (e.g., walking, cycling) or 40 minutes of vigorous activity (e.g., running, HIIT). This schedule ensures you're hitting all 12 categories while also balancing your meals and workouts throughout the day!

3. Dr. Eric Berg – The Role of Ketosis and Insulin Control

Dr. Berg advocates for low-carb and ketogenic diets to combat insulin resistance and promote fat loss. He highlights the importance of nutrient-dense meals to sustain energy and health.

Dr. Berg's Key Dietary Principles

- **Low-Carb, High-Fat (LCHF) Diet**
  Prioritize healthy fats while significantly reducing carbohydrate intake to encourage fat-burning (ketosis).
  Examples: Avocado, olive oil, butter, nuts, seeds, fatty fish.

- **Intermittent Fasting (IF)**
  Incorporate eating windows (e.g., 16:8((Fasting period: Eating window) or OMAD - One Meal A Day) to stabilize insulin and promote autophagy.

- **Nutrient-Dense Foods**
  Focus on foods rich in vitamins, minerals, and antioxidants to support overall health.

Examples: Leafy greens, cruciferous vegetables, eggs, grass-fed meats.

- **Adequate Protein**
  Consume moderate protein to avoid overstimulating insulin while maintaining muscle mass.
  Examples: Chicken, fish, eggs, cheese, and tofu.

- **Electrolyte Balance**
  Support hydration and mineral levels (sodium, potassium, magnesium) during ketosis.
  Examples: Himalayan salt, leafy greens, bone broth.

- **Avoid Refined Sugars and Processed Carbs**
  Eliminate high-glycemic foods to prevent blood sugar spikes and crashes.

4. Dr. Mark Hyman – Functional Medicine and Food as Medicine

Dr. Hyman champions the transformative role of food in preventing, managing, and even reversing chronic illnesses. By combining functional medicine principles with personalized nutrition, he emphasizes anti-inflammatory, nutrient-dense diets to promote optimal health. He also highlights magnesium's diverse forms and benefits, often calling it the ultimate antidote to stress.

Magnesium: A powerful relaxation mineral		
Constipation	Magnesium Citrate	Draws water into the intestines
Stress & Sleep	Magnesium Glycinate	Calms the nervous system
Muscle Pain	Magnesium Malate	Aids muscle recovery and reduces fatigue.
Indigestion	Magnesium Oxide	Acts as an antacid, neutralizing stomach acid
Heart Health	Magnesium Taurate	Supports heart rhythm and blood pressure regulation.
Cognition	Magnesium L-threonate	Enhances brain function and memory by crossing the blood-brain barrier

Did you know that soaking in a hot bath with <u>Epsom salts</u> (magnesium sulfate) is an excellent way to boost your magnesium levels?

The Five Key Biomarkers for Metabolic Health

Biomarker	Why It Matters	How to Optimize
Blood Sugar Levels	Indicates glucose metabolism; high levels can lead to insulin resistance and type 2 diabetes.	- Diet: Whole foods, low-GI carbs, high-fiber foods. - Exercise: Aerobic + strength training. - Timing: Avoid late eating, try time-restricted eating. - Supplements: Berberine, chromium (consult doctor).
Triglycerides	High levels linked to insulin resistance and cardiovascular risk.	- Diet: Reduce refined carbs, sugar, focus on omega-3s. - Alcohol: Limit or avoid. - Exercise: Regular cardio.
HDL Cholesterol	Removes excess cholesterol, protects against cardiovascular disease.	- Healthy Fats: Omega-3s, monounsaturated fats (avocado, olive oil). - Exercise: High-intensity interval training (HIIT).
Waist-to-Hip Ratio	High ratio signals visceral fat, linked to inflammation and chronic disease.	- Diet: Anti-inflammatory, whole foods, lean proteins. - Exercise: Strength training + cardio. - Stress Management: Meditation, yoga.

Biomarker	Why It Matters	How to Optimize
Blood Pressure	High blood pressure increases risk of heart disease, stroke, and kidney issues.	- Sodium & Potassium Balance: Reduce sodium, increase potassium-rich foods (bananas, spinach). - Exercise: Aerobic activities. - Weight Management: Even small losses help. - Relaxation Techniques: Box breathing, meditation. - Hydration: Stay hydrated.

5. Dr. Hiromi Shinya – The Enzyme Secret

Dr. Hiromi Shinya, a renowned gastroenterologist, revolutionized digestive health with his enzyme-focused dietary principles. He emphasizes the role of enzyme-rich foods in enhancing gut function, boosting vitality, and promoting overall well-being.

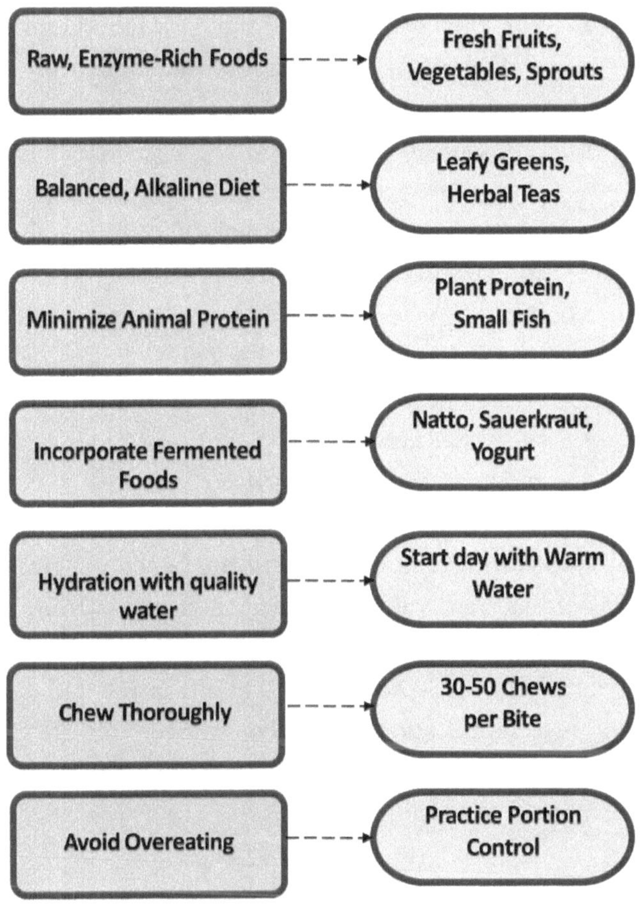

Dr. Shinya's Key Dietary Principles

- Prioritize uncooked, natural foods to preserve enzymes vital for digestion and cellular repair.
- Favor alkaline-forming foods to maintain pH balance and reduce inflammation.

- Limit intake of red meat and dairy to reduce the burden on the digestive system and prevent toxin accumulation.
- Drink plenty of mineral-rich, purified water to support enzyme activity and detoxification.
- Chew food well to activate enzymes in saliva and enhance nutrient absorption.
- Practice portion control to ease digestive strain and prevent enzyme depletion. Follow the "Hara Hachi Bu" principle—eat until 80% full.
- Boost gut health with probiotic-rich foods that enhance microbiome diversity.

6. Dr. Verena Tan – Cracking the Glycemic Code

Dr. Verena Tan, a leading expert in glycemic control, emphasizes the role of low-GI (glycemic index) foods in stabilizing blood sugar levels. Her research and dietary recommendations focus on preventing energy crashes, reducing sugar cravings, and supporting long-term metabolic health.

Dr. Tan's Key Dietary Principles

Prioritize Low-GI Foods

- Opt for foods that release glucose slowly to maintain stable energy levels and reduce insulin spikes.
- Examples: Whole grains like quinoa, rolled oats, lentils, and sweet potatoes.

Balance Your Meals

- Combine low-GI carbs with protein, healthy fats, and fiber to create balanced meals that curb cravings.
- Examples: Grilled salmon with quinoa and steamed vegetables or hummus with whole-grain pita and a side salad.

Choose Natural Sugars

- Replace refined sugars with natural sweeteners in moderation.
- Examples: Use honey, dates, or fruits like berries and apples for sweetness.

Incorporate Fiber-Rich Foods

- Boost dietary fiber to slow digestion, enhance satiety, and improve glycemic control.
- Examples: Chia seeds, flaxseeds, leafy greens, and legumes.

Mind Your Portions

- Keep portions of even low-GI foods in check to prevent overloading the system with glucose.
- Tip: Use the plate method—fill half with vegetables, a quarter with protein, and a quarter with low-GI carbs.

Snack Smart

- Choose low-GI snacks that sustain energy without triggering spikes.

- Examples: Handful of nuts, boiled eggs, or Greek yogurt with fresh fruit.

7. Dr. Tim Spector – The Microbiome Whisperer

Dr. Tim Spector, a renowned epidemiologist and microbiome expert, emphasizes the transformative power of dietary diversity to nurture gut health. He highlights how a thriving gut microbiome influences immunity, metabolism, mood, and overall well-being.

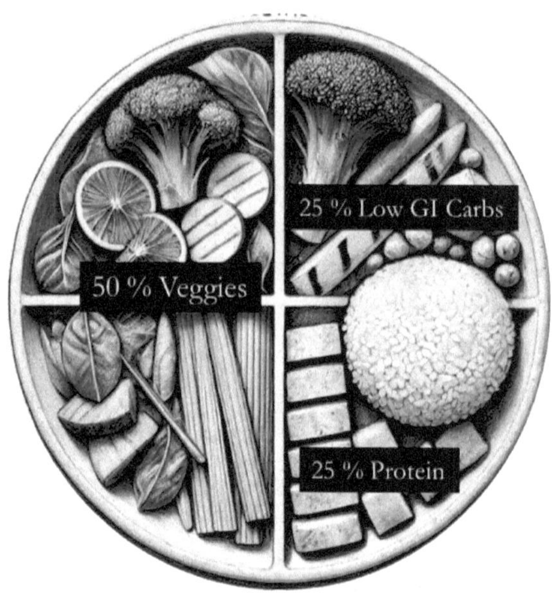

Dr. Spector's Key Dietary Principles

Embrace Dietary Diversity

- Aim for at least 30 different plant-based foods per week to support a rich and diverse microbiome.

- Examples: Vegetables, fruits, whole grains, legumes, nuts, seeds, and herbs.

Prioritize Fermented Foods
- Incorporate probiotic-rich foods to introduce beneficial bacteria.
- Examples: Yogurt, kefir, kimchi, sauerkraut, and miso.

Feed Your Microbiome with Fiber
- Include prebiotic fibers to nourish gut bacteria and promote their growth.
- Examples: Garlic, onions, leeks, bananas, and asparagus.

Limit Ultra-Processed Foods
- Avoid foods high in additives, sugar, and unhealthy fats, which can harm gut diversity.
- Examples: Replace processed snacks with whole food alternatives like nuts or fruit.

Experiment with Polyphenols
- Add polyphenol-rich foods to boost gut bacteria diversity and reduce inflammation.
- Examples: Dark chocolate, berries, green tea, and extra virgin olive oil.

Explore Personalized Nutrition
- Recognize that gut health varies among individuals, and tailor dietary choices accordingly.

- Tip: Use microbiome testing tools or keep a food diary to discover your optimal gut-friendly foods.

8. Rujuta Diwekar – Ancient Wisdom, Modern Nutrition

Rujuta Diwekar, a leading Indian nutritionist, champions the timeless wisdom of eating local, seasonal, and traditional foods. Her holistic approach bridges heritage with modern lifestyles, promoting health, sustainability, and mindful eating.

Diwekar's Key Dietary Principles

Eat Local and Seasonal

- Consume foods grown in your region and suited to the current season for optimal nutrition and digestion.
- Examples: Mangoes in summer, leafy greens in winter, millets in monsoon.

Respect Traditional Recipes

- Celebrate the culinary wisdom of your ancestors by preparing meals using age-old techniques and local ingredients.
- Examples: Ghee-laden rotis, coconut-based curries, fermented idlis.

Avoid Packaged and Processed Foods

- Steer clear of foods with long ingredient lists and artificial additives.

- Tip: Opt for fresh, home-cooked meals over pre-packaged alternatives.

Embrace Whole Foods
- Choose unrefined foods over polished or processed versions.
- Examples: Brown rice over white rice, jaggery over refined sugar.

Follow the "Rule of Portion and Timing"
- Eat according to your body's hunger signals and align meals with your daily activity levels.
- Tip: Breakfast like a king, lunch like a prince, and dinner like a pauper.

Incorporate Ghee and Traditional Fats
- Use natural fats like ghee and coconut oil in moderation for their health benefits.
- Example: A dollop of ghee on rice enhances both flavor and digestion.

Hydrate Smartly
- Stay hydrated but avoid overloading on packaged beverages.
- Tip: Start your day with a glass of warm water or herbal tea.

9. Dr. Satoshi Sasaki – Sodium-Potassium Balance

Dr. Satoshi Sasaki, a renowned expert in cardiovascular

health, emphasizes the crucial role of balancing sodium (Na) and potassium (K) intake for maintaining optimal heart health and regulating blood pressure. His research highlights how this balance is vital for preventing hypertension, stroke, and other cardiovascular diseases.

Dr. Satoshi Sasaki's Heart-Healthy Blueprint

Sodium-Potassium Harmony: The Heart's Balancing Act

- Striking the right balance between sodium and potassium is key to controlling blood pressure and preventing heart issues.
- Pro Tip: Reduce salt and load up on potassium-rich foods like bananas and avocados.

Whole Foods, Whole Health

- Processed foods often tip the sodium scale, while fresh options keep the balance in check.
- Pro Tip: Swap packaged snacks for vibrant veggies, fruits, legumes, and grains.

Ditch the Salt Shaker

- Too much salt spells trouble for your heart, but natural seasonings make meals flavorful and healthy.
- Pro Tip: Jazz up your dishes with herbs, spices, lemon, or a splash of vinegar.

Potassium-Packed Plates

- Potassium works wonders to counter sodium's effects and keep your heart thriving.
- Pro Tip: Add sweet potatoes, spinach, or creamy avocados to your daily menu.

Know Your Numbers

- Regular blood pressure checks are your compass to heart health.
- Pro Tip: Keep your readings near 120/80 mmHg for a steady, strong heart.

10. Dr. Megan Rossi – Prebiotics and Probiotics for Gut Health

Dr. Megan Rossi, known as "The Gut Health Doctor," is a leading expert in microbiome health. She emphasizes the importance of prebiotics and probiotics in nurturing gut health, improving digestion, and boosting immunity. Her work highlights how a diverse gut microbiome is essential for overall health, affecting everything from mood to metabolism.

Dr. Megan Rossi's Gut Health Playbook

Prebiotics: Feed the Good Guys

- Fuel your gut with non-digestible fibers that nurture beneficial bacteria.
- Pro Tip: Toss in onions, garlic, asparagus, and bananas to supercharge your microbiome.

Probiotics: Populate with the Best

- Replenish your gut's army of friendly bacteria for optimal digestion.

- Pro Tip: Enjoy yogurt, kefir, kimchi, or a fizzy kombucha for a probiotic punch.

Gut Diversity: A Symphony of Bacteria

- A diverse microbiome equals a resilient digestive system.
- Pro Tip: Mix it up with fiber-rich fruits, veggies, whole grains, nuts, and legumes in every meal.

Fermented Foods: Nature's Probiotic Powerhouses

- Fermented delights enhance digestion and immune strength while bridging the gut-brain connection.
- Pro Tip: Miso soup, tempeh wraps, or tangy pickles are tasty ways to nourish your gut.

Fiber: The Gut's Favorite Fuel

- Both prebiotics and probiotics thrive on fiber for a balanced microbiome.
- Pro Tip: Aim for 30 grams of plant-based fiber daily from colorful plates filled with whole, fresh foods.

Building Your Personal Nutrition Plan

Here's how to synthesize these insights:

1. **Experiment and Observe:** Try different eating patterns (e.g., intermittent fasting or plant-based meals) and track how you feel.

2. **Balance Science and Tradition:** Combine expert-backed principles with the cultural foods you love.

3. **Stay Flexible**: Nutrition is dynamic. Adapt as needed.

Practical Takeaways for a Personalized Nutrition Plan

- Adopt a predominantly plant-based diet, complemented by occasional fish.
- Avoid overeating, especially late at night.
- Use Fast Mimicking Diet (FMD) or intermittent fasting to reset your system and optimize cellular health.
- Prioritize nutrient density and minimize sugar for sustainable energy and metabolic stability.
- Maintain consistent meal times to support circadian rhythms.

Foods That Are "Eating You Up"

Don't let your plate dig your grave—choose foods that fuel you, not ones that consume you!

1. **Excess Salt:** Causes calcium depletion, increasing the risk of osteoporosis.

2. **Refined Sugar:** Promotes inflammation and oxidative stress, accelerating aging and metabolic dysfunction.

3. **Trans Fats:** Found in processed snacks, disrupts cell membranes and increases the risk of heart disease.

4. **Excess Alcohol:** Impairs liver function, depletes nutrients like B vitamins, and contributes to oxidative stress.

5. **Artificial Sweeteners:** Disrupt gut microbiota, potentially causing metabolic and digestive issues.

6. **Fried Foods:** High in advanced glycation end products (AGEs), which promote inflammation and oxidative damage.

7. **Processed Meats:** High in sodium and nitrates, linked to increased inflammation and cancer risk.

8. **Refined Oils (e.g., Soybean, Corn, Canola):** High in omega-6 fatty acids, fueling inflammation and disrupting omega-3 balance.

9. **Excess Caffeine:** Depletes magnesium and disrupts sleep, leading to stress and hormonal imbalances.

10. **Soft Drinks:** Acidic and sugary, contributing to tooth enamel erosion, bone mineral loss, and insulin spikes.

11. **White Bread and Refined Carbs:** Spikes blood sugar, leading to insulin resistance and fat storage.

12. **Excess Dairy:** May contribute to inflammation and acne in sensitive individuals.

13. **Packaged/Instant Foods:** High in preservatives and additives, which can stress detoxification systems in the liver.

14. **Charred/Grilled Meats:** Contains heterocyclic amines (HCAs) and polycyclic aromatic hydrocarbons (PAHs), linked to cancer.

15. **High-Mercury Fish (e.g., Tuna, Swordfish):** Accumulated mercury damages nervous system and brain function.

16. **Artificial Food Coloring:** Linked to hyperactivity and potential toxicity in sensitive individuals.

Daily Intake Guidelines

Here's a simple and practical list to guide your daily nutrition intake:

1. **Protein:**
   - Goal: 0.8–1.2 grams per kilogram of body weight.
   - Example: If you weigh 70 kg, aim for 56–84 grams of protein daily.
   - Sources: Eggs, chicken, lentils, tofu, fish, nuts.

2. **Carbohydrates:**
   - Goal: 45–65% of daily caloric intake, prioritizing complex carbs.
   - Example: For a 2000-calorie diet, 225–325 grams of carbs.
   - Sources: Whole grains, legumes, starchy vegetables.

3. **Healthy Fats:**
   - Goal: 20–35% of daily caloric intake.
   - Example: For a 2000-calorie diet, 44–77 grams of fat.
   - Sources: Olive oil, nuts, seeds, avocados.
4. **Sugar:**
   - Goal: Less than 10% of daily caloric intake (preferably <25 grams).
   - Example: Avoid added sugars; enjoy natural sugars in fruits.
5. **Salt (Sodium):**
   - Goal: <1 teaspoon (2,300 mg) daily; ideally 1,500 mg for optimal heart health.
   - Tip: Avoid salty snacks and processed foods.
6. **Fiber:**
   - Goal: 25–30 grams daily.
   - Sources: Vegetables, fruits, whole grains, legumes.
7. **Water:**
   - Goal: 2–3 liters daily (varies by activity level and climate).
   - Tip: Drink regularly throughout the day, even when not thirsty.
8. **Calcium:**
   - Goal: 1,000–1,200 mg daily.
   - Sources: Dairy, fortified plant milk, leafy greens.
9. **Iron:**
   - Goal: 8–18 mg daily (higher for women of

reproductive age).
- Sources: Red meat, spinach, beans, fortified cereals.

10. **Vitamin D:**
- Goal: 600–800 IU daily.
- Sources: Sunlight, fatty fish, fortified foods.

11. **Omega-3 Fatty Acids:**
- Goal: 250–500 mg of EPA/DHA daily.
- Sources: Salmon, mackerel, walnuts, flaxseeds.

12. **Fruits and Vegetables:**
- Goal: At least 5 servings (400–500 grams) daily.
- Tip: Aim for a rainbow of colors to maximize nutrients.

Bioactive Power List: Fuel Your Body, Elevate Your Life!

Bioactive compounds are natural chemical substances found in foods that promote health and prevent disease by interacting with the body's biological processes.

1. **Urolithin A** – Boost your mitochondria, your body's power plants!
   Sources: Pomegranates, almonds, walnuts, raspberries, blackberries.

2. **Curcumin** – Defend against inflammation, naturally.
   Sources: Turmeric, yellow mustard.

3. **Resveratrol** – Toast to heart health and longevity.
Sources: Grapes, red wine, peanuts, blueberries, mulberries.

4. **Quercetin** – Charge up your immunity like a pro!
Sources: Onions, apples, berries, capers, citrus fruits.

5. **EGCG (**Epigallocatechin gallate**)** – Sharpen focus and burn calories!
Sources: Green tea, white tea, black tea, guava leaves.

6. **Lycopene** – Protect your skin and glow with UV defense.
Sources: Tomatoes, watermelon, pink grapefruit, papaya, red peppers.

7. **Anthocyanins** – Fight oxidative stress with vibrant colors.
Sources: Blueberries, blackberries, cherries, eggplants, purple cabbage.

8. **Berberine** – Balance your gut and glucose levels.
Sources: Barberry, goldenseal, Oregon grape, tree turmeric, Phellodendron.

9. **Sulforaphane** – Detox like a wellness guru!
Sources: Broccoli, Brussels sprouts, kale, cauliflower, mustard greens.

10. **Ellagic Acid** – Fight cancer with nature's bounty.
Sources: Strawberries, raspberries, pomegranates, walnuts, pecans.

11. **Astaxanthin** – Glow from the inside out!
Sources: Salmon, shrimp, krill, trout, microalgae.

12. **Catechins** – Boost heart health and sustain energy.
    Sources: Green tea, black tea, cocoa, apples, pears, dark chocolate.

13. **Flavonoids** – Brighten your brain and lower inflammation.
    Sources: Dark chocolate, berries, red wine, citrus fruits.

14. **Theobromine** – Improve mood and circulation with a cocoa hug!
    Sources: Dark chocolate, cocoa powder, cacao nibs.

15. **Polyphenols** – Be an oxidative stress warrior!
    Sources: Dark chocolate, olive oil, green tea.

16. **Beta-Glucans** – Supercharge your immunity.
    Sources: Oats, mushrooms (shiitake, reishi), barley, yeast.

17. **Lutein** – Protect your vision, bite by bite.
    Sources: Spinach, kale, egg yolks, zucchini, peas.

18. **Zeaxanthin** – Keep your eyes sparkling and strong!
    Sources: Corn, yellow peppers, goji berries, eggs.

19. **Ginsenosides** – Stress relief meets energy boost.
    Sources: Ginseng varieties (Panax, Siberian, American).

20. **Genistein** – Balance hormones for a strong, happy you.
    Sources: Soybeans, chickpeas, lentils, fava beans.

21. **Omega-3 Fatty Acids** – Stay sharp and inflammation-free.
    Sources: Fatty fish, flaxseeds, walnuts, chia seeds.

22. **Fisetin** – Age gracefully, stay vibrant.
    Sources: Strawberries, apples, persimmons, cucumbers.

23. **Hydroxytyrosol** – Heart health in every olive drizzle.
    Sources: Olive oil, black tea, white wine.

Start incorporating these wonders and watch your health soar!

The Hand-rule Approach

Ensures balanced portions without the need for scales or measuring cups.

Daily Food Portions Using the Hand Rule		
Nuts & Seeds	A handful (about 1 ounce)	Almonds, walnuts, or sunflower seeds for healthy fats and protein.
Protein	A palm-sized portion (3–4 ounces for women, 4–6 ounces for men)	Chicken, fish, tofu, or lentils to meet daily protein needs.
Vegetables	Two open hands cupped together (about 2 cups)	Leafy greens, broccoli, or bell peppers for fiber and vitamins.
Fruits	A fist-sized portion (about 1 cup)	Apples, berries, or oranges for natural sweetness and antioxidants.
Carbohydrates (Whole Grains or Starches)	A fist-sized portion (about 1 cup)	Quinoa, brown rice, or sweet potatoes for sustained energy.
Fats (Oils or Butters)	Thumb-sized portion (about 1 tablespoon)	Olive oil, ghee, or nut butter for essential fatty acids.
Dairy (if included)	Two thumb-sized portions (about 1 ounce each)	Cheese, yogurt, or milk for calcium and probiotics.
Snacks (e.g., Dark Chocolate)	A thumb-sized portion (1–2 small squares)	Opt for 70% cocoa or higher for health benefits.

Closing Thoughts:

You've journeyed through a wealth of insights, but there's still much more ahead. Take a moment, grab a refreshing glass of water, and hydrate—because a well-fueled mind is the key to absorbing what's next!

Benefits of Infused Water

Infused water, created by adding fruits, vegetables, herbs, or spices to water, offers a flavorful and nutrient-enhanced alternative to plain water. Here's a breakdown of its benefits backed by scientific insights:

1. **Improved Hydration**
   - Staying hydrated can improve energy levels and cognitive performance by up to 14%, especially in mildly dehydrated individuals.
   - Flavored water can encourage higher water intake, helping meet the recommended 2.7–3.7 liters/day for adults.

2. **Enhanced Antioxidant Intake**
   - Fruits like citrus, berries, and herbs (e.g., mint) release antioxidants such as vitamin C and polyphenols into water, providing up to 20–30% of their total content.
   - These antioxidants combat oxidative stress and support skin health, immunity, and overall well-being.

3. **Weight Management**

- Drinking infused water before meals can reduce calorie intake by ~13% (approximately 75–90 calories per meal).
- It acts as a natural appetite suppressant and supports fat metabolism.

4. Improved Digestive Health

- Ingredients like ginger and lemon in infused water can increase digestive enzyme activity by 20–25%.
- It promotes smoother digestion and reduces bloating.

5. Enhanced Detoxification

- Certain infusions, such as cucumber and mint, can boost natural detoxification processes, enhancing kidney filtration rates by 10–15%.
- Supports liver and kidney function for efficient toxin elimination.

6. Improved Skin Health

- Regular hydration with infused water can improve skin elasticity and hydration by 11–18%.
- Antioxidants in the infusions help reduce signs of aging and promote a radiant complexion.

7. Reduced Sugar Intake

- Switching from sugary drinks to infused water can reduce sugar consumption by 30–50 grams daily, cutting up to 200 calories.

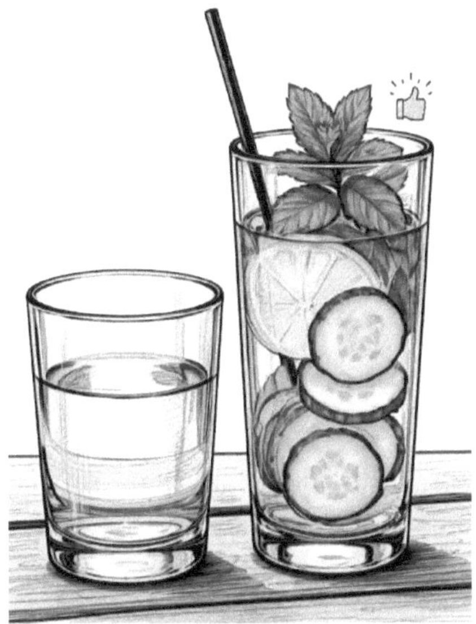

- Helps prevent weight gain, insulin resistance, and type 2 diabetes.

8. Electrolyte Support

- Adding citrus fruits or coconut water provides natural electrolytes, improving rehydration by up to 16% compared to plain water.
- Beneficial for post-exercise recovery and preventing dehydration.

Top Ingredients and Their Benefits

- **Lemon:** High in vitamin C (30–40 mg per lemon); boosts immunity and collagen production.

- **Cucumber:** Contains silica; supports skin health and hydration.
- **Mint:** Contains menthol; improves digestion and reduces bloating.
- **Berries:** Rich in anthocyanins; reduce inflammation and support heart health.
- **Ginger:** Contains gingerol; alleviates nausea and enhances metabolism.

Infused water combines hydration with added health benefits, contributing to improved digestion, weight management, detoxification, and more. By integrating natural, nutrient-rich ingredients, infused water offers a scientifically backed, calorie-free alternative to sugary beverages for enhanced overall health.

9 SUPER FOODS

"Your diet is a bank account. Good food choices are good investments"

— *Bethenny Frankel*

Superfoods are nutrient-dense foods offering significant health benefits, supporting everything from brain function to cellular repair. Incorporating them into your diet can optimize health and enhance your biohacking potential. Below is a comprehensive list of superfoods categorized by their specific benefits and properties.

1. Brain-Boosting Superfoods

These foods enhance cognitive function, memory, and focus, making them essential for mental clarity:

- Dark Chocolate: Rich in flavonoids that improve blood flow to the brain, enhancing memory and cognition, and containing mood-boosting compounds like theobromine.

- Blueberries: Packed with antioxidants, especially anthocyanins, that support memory, learning, and protection against age-related decline.
- Turmeric: Contains curcumin, an anti-inflammatory compound that boosts brain-derived neurotrophic factor (BDNF), crucial for neural growth and cognitive function.
- Ginkgo Biloba: Improves memory and focus by increasing blood flow to the brain.
- Ashwagandha: A powerful adaptogen that reduces stress and enhances cognitive performance.
- Brahmi (Bacopa Monnieri): Promotes cognitive function, memory, and mental clarity. Fosters dendrite and synapse growth, improving communication between brain cells while providing antioxidant protection.

2. Heart-Healthy Superfoods

These foods promote cardiovascular health by lowering blood pressure and improving circulation:

- Macadamia Nuts: High in monounsaturated fats and magnesium, reducing cholesterol and inflammation.
- Olives & Olive Oil: Rich in oleic acid, offering anti-inflammatory benefits and lowering heart

disease risk.

- Chia Seeds: Provide omega-3 fatty acids, fiber, and antioxidants to support heart health.
- Salmon (Wild-caught): An excellent source of omega-3s, reducing inflammation and promoting circulation.
- Beets: High in nitrates that enhance blood flow and lower blood pressure.

3. Immune-Boosting Superfoods

These strengthen the immune system and enhance disease resistance:

- Garlic: Contains antimicrobial properties and boosts immune response.
- Ginger: Rich in gingerol, it reduces inflammation and strengthens immunity.
- Citrus Fruits: Packed with vitamin C, they enhance immunity and skin health.
- Elderberries: Provide antioxidants and vitamin C to fight infections and flu.
- Mushrooms (Reishi, Shiitake, Maitake): Contain beta-glucans that support cellular health and reduce inflammation.

4. Anti-Inflammatory Superfoods

These reduce chronic inflammation, a root cause of many diseases:

- Turmeric: With curcumin as a key anti-inflammatory agent.

- Berries: Rich in anthocyanins to combat oxidative stress.
- Leafy Greens: Kale and spinach reduce inflammation with vitamins and phytonutrients.
- Avocados: Provide healthy fats and inflammation-fighting compounds.
- Green Tea: Contains EGCG, a powerful antioxidant.

5. Energy-Enhancing Superfoods

These foods sustain energy levels and enhance physical performance:

- Avocados: Offer slow-releasing energy through healthy fats.
- Sweet Potatoes: Provide complex carbs and beta-carotene for metabolism.
- Bananas: High in potassium for quick energy and electrolyte balance.
- Oats: Deliver slow-digesting carbs for steady energy.
- Maca Root: Boosts stamina and endurance naturally.

6. Gut-Health Superfoods

These promote a healthy microbiome and improve digestion:

- Yogurt: Packed with probiotics for digestive health.

- Kefir: A fermented drink that balances gut bacteria.
- Sauerkraut: Provides probiotics and fiber for digestion.
- Kimchi: Contains anti-inflammatory probiotics.
- Apple Cider Vinegar: Enhances digestion and detoxification.

7. Skin-Nourishing Superfoods

These enhance skin health, elasticity, and protection:
- Avocados: Rich in fats and antioxidants for skin hydration.
- Carrots: High in beta-carotene to improve skin turnover.
- Tomatoes: Contain lycopene to guard against UV damage.
- Nuts: Offer vitamin E for hydration and protection.
- Coconut Oil: Moisturizes and reduces inflammation.

8. Detoxifying Superfoods

These support the body's natural detox processes:
- Lemon: Flushes toxins and aids liver function.
- Cilantro: Binds heavy metals for removal.
- Beets: Rich in antioxidants for liver health.
- Dandelion Greens: Cleanse the liver and kidneys.

- Parsley: Acts as a natural diuretic for toxin removal.

9. Bone-Health Superfoods

These strengthen bones and support skeletal health:
- Leafy Greens: Provide calcium and vitamin K for bone density.
- Salmon: Enhances calcium absorption with omega-3s and vitamin D.
- Tofu: A plant-based source of calcium and protein.
- Chia Seeds: Boost bone strength with calcium and magnesium.
- Almonds: Rich in nutrients to combat osteoporosis.

Minerals: The Unsung heroes of Health and Vitality

Minerals are essential nutrients that play a critical role in maintaining overall health and well-being. They contribute to over 300 biochemical reactions in the body, supporting processes like energy production, bone formation, nerve function, and immune defense. For instance, calcium, which constitutes 1.5% of an average adult's body weight, is vital for strong bones and teeth, while magnesium regulates over 600 enzymatic reactions, influencing muscle function and sleep quality. Trace minerals like zinc and selenium, though required in microgram quantities, are crucial for DNA synthesis and antioxidant defense. Without adequate mineral intake, risks of chronic conditions such as osteoporosis, anemia, and cardiovascular disease significantly increase.

Here are mineral-based wellness hacks to incorporate into your routine:

1. **Magnesium Relaxation**: Soak in an Epsom salt (magnesium sulfate) bath to relieve muscle tension and stress.
2. **Zinc for Immunity**: Suck on zinc lozenges at the first sign of a cold to boost immune response.
3. **Iron Absorption**: Pair iron-rich foods (like spinach or lentils) with vitamin C (like citrus fruits) to enhance absorption.
4. **Calcium for Bones**: Add a pinch of ground eggshells (rich in calcium) to smoothies for stronger bones.
5. **Selenium Boost**: Eat just two Brazil nuts a day to meet your selenium needs and support thyroid health.
6. **Potassium Hydration**: Snack on bananas or avocados to maintain electrolyte balance and prevent muscle cramps.
7. **Copper Glow**: Use copper-infused water bottles to benefit from trace amounts of copper, which supports collagen production.
8. **Silica for Hair and Nails**: Incorporate horsetail tea into your diet for silica, promoting stronger hair and nails.

"You can trace every sickness, every disease, and every ailment to a mineral deficiency."
–Linus Pauling

(Two-time Nobel Prize winner)

9. **Iodine for Thyroid Health**: Include seaweed like nori or kelp in your meals to boost iodine levels.
10. **Chromium for Blood Sugar**: Add brewer's yeast to foods to improve insulin sensitivity and stabilize blood sugar levels.
11. **Sulfur Detox**: Incorporate sulfur-rich foods like garlic, onions, and cruciferous vegetables for detoxification.
12. **Boron for Bones**: Add prunes to your diet for boron, which supports bone health and hormone regulation.
13. **Manganese for Joints**: Sprinkle ground cloves or cinnamon on your meals to benefit from manganese for joint health.
14. **Fluoride for Teeth**: Drink green tea, which contains natural fluoride to strengthen teeth and fight decay.
15. **Phosphorus for Energy**: Eat sunflower seeds to boost phosphorus intake, crucial for energy production.
16. **Sodium Balance**: Add Himalayan pink salt to your meals for a natural source of trace minerals and sodium.
17. **Magnesium Oil**: Apply magnesium oil directly to your skin for faster absorption to relieve aches and improve sleep.
18. **Lithium Calm**: Drink mineral water rich in lithium to help reduce stress and stabilize mood.
19. **Molybdenum for Detox**: Eat lentils or kidney beans to support your body's detox pathways with

molybdenum.

20. **Vanadium for Glucose**: Add black pepper to your diet, a natural source of vanadium, to aid in glucose metabolism.

Closing Thoughts: Incorporating Super-foods for Total Wellness

Adding a variety of these superfoods into your diet can enhance energy, strengthen immunity, and optimize your body's natural functions. From boosting brain power to fortifying bone health, each superfood offers unique benefits for your biohacking journey.

10 BRAIN FUEL

"Your brain is the most energy-hungry organ—
fuel it wisely, and it will power your greatest
ideas."

— *Dr. Caroline Leaf*

Our brains are powerful yet underutilized tools, often constrained by the mental barriers we impose on ourselves. To unlock their full potential, we must harness the trifecta of mindset, motivation, and methods. With the right strategies, we can rewrite limiting beliefs, ignite a thirst for knowledge, and employ effective techniques to foster a limitless mind. This chapter dives into practical strategies for breaking mental barriers and fueling your brain for peak performance.

Memory Magic: Unlocking the Power of Retention

Memory is not a gift reserved for the few—it's a skill anyone can cultivate. Here are methods to boost retention:

1. **Visualization**: Transform abstract information into vivid mental images. Picture numbers as vibrant objects or historical events as movie scenes.
2. **Storytelling**: Weave facts into engaging narratives. For example, remember grocery items by crafting a funny story linking each item.
3. **Mnemonic Devices**: Use acronyms, rhymes, or chunking to group and recall information effortlessly.

Practice these techniques daily, and watch as your memory evolves into an effortless superpower.

Read Like the Wind: Speed Reading Secrets

Speed reading isn't just about reading faster; it's about reading smarter. *"Your brain is like a muscle. The more you use it, the stronger it gets"* – Jim Kwik

- **Minimize Subvocalization**: Silence the inner voice that reads aloud in your mind.
- **Use a Visual Pacer**: Guide your eyes with your finger or a pen to maintain focus.
- **Chunk Words Together**: Instead of reading word by word, grasp entire phrases in one glance.
- **Preview the Text**: Scan headings, subheadings, and key points to understand the structure before diving in.

These methods will help you devour books and articles in record time while retaining key insights.

Benefits of Watching Content at 2x Speed

- **Efficiency:** Consuming videos or podcasts at double speed allows you to cover more content in less time, enhancing productivity.
- **Retention Boost:** Faster playback keeps your brain actively engaged, reducing distractions and improving focus. Studies suggest that people retain information equally well at 1.5x or 2x speeds compared to normal playback.
- **Cognitive Flexibility**: Regularly processing information at higher speeds trains your brain to think and analyze more quickly, enhancing cognitive agility.
- **Reduced Boredom:** Accelerated playback can make slow-paced content more engaging, maintaining interest in longer educational materials.

Recharge Your Brain: The Science of Self-Care

Optimal brain performance depends on physical and mental well-being. Embrace these self-care strategies:

1. **Sleep Deeply**: Prioritize 7-9 hours of restorative sleep. Deep sleep consolidates memories and clears toxins from the brain.
2. **Exercise Regularly**: Aerobic activities increase blood flow and stimulate the release of brain-derived neurotrophic factor (BDNF),

enhancing neurogenesis.

3. **Manage Stress**: Practice mindfulness, yoga, or breathing techniques like box breathing to calm your mind and sharpen focus.

4. **Fuel Your Brain**: Eat nutrient-rich foods such as blueberries, walnuts, and salmon. Avoid sugar crashes by maintaining balanced glucose levels.

Breaking Mental Barriers: Rewriting Your Belief System

To break mental barriers, we must first identify and question self-limiting beliefs. Follow these steps:

- **Acknowledge Your Beliefs**: Reflect on phrases like "I'm not smart enough" or "I'm too old to learn."
- **Challenge the Narrative**: Replace negativity with empowering beliefs like "I'm capable" and "It's never too late."
- **Rewire Through Action**: Take small, consistent steps to prove your new beliefs. Success reinforces confidence and dismantles old constraints.

"Fuel your brain like a Ferrari, not a food truck."

– Anonymous

Biohacks for Brain Fuel

Maximize cognitive performance with these science-backed strategies:

1. **Intermittent Fasting**: Enhance focus and mental clarity through fasting protocols like 16/8.
2. **Brainwave Entrainment**: Use binaural beats to stimulate desired brainwave states (e.g., alpha waves for relaxation).
3. **Nootropics**: Explore natural supplements like Lion's Mane Mushroom and Bacopa Monnieri to boost memory and focus.
4. **Cold Showers**: Sharpen your mind by triggering norepinephrine production with cold exposure.
5. **Mindful Breathing**: Techniques like 4-7-8 breathing enhance oxygen flow to the brain and reduce stress.

Experiment with these biohacks to discover what resonates with your unique brain chemistry.

Incorporating Binaural Beats into Your Productivity Routine

Choose the Right Frequency Each brainwave frequency enhances a specific mental state:

- **Alpha (8–14 Hz)**: Calm focus and creative flow—ideal for brainstorming and relaxed work.

- **Beta (14–30 Hz)**: Active focus and concentration—perfect for problem-solving and logical tasks.
- **Gamma (30–100 Hz)**: Enhanced cognition and learning—best for deep thinking.

Best Time to Listen

- **Morning (9–11 AM)**: Use Beta waves for deep work.
- **Afternoon Slump (2–4 PM)**: Switch to Alpha waves to regain calm focus.
- **Creative Work**: Theta waves (4–8 Hz) support idea generation.

Tools for Binaural Beats

- **Brain.fm**: Focus-enhancing soundscapes.
- **MyNoise**: Customizable tones.
- **Spotify/YouTube**: Search "Binaural Beats for Focus."
- **Headspace/Calm**: Guided sessions with embedded beats.

Productivity Ritual with Binaural Beats Pair beats with the Pomodoro technique:
Combine with Other Techniques

- **Environment**: Use noise-cancelling headphones.
- **Mindful Breaks**: Listen to Alpha waves to reset.
- **Task-Specific Playlists**:

> Writing: Alpha waves.
> Problem-solving: Beta waves.
> Learning: Gamma waves.

Duration and Volume

- Listen for 15–45 minutes at 50–60% volume.
- Avoid sessions over 1 hour to prevent fatigue.

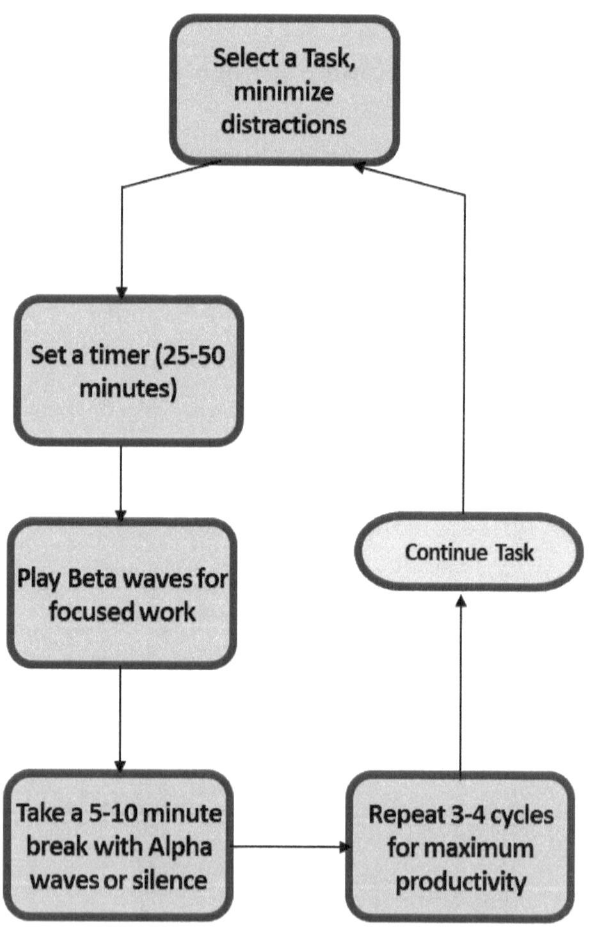

Brain Foods: A Fusion of Modern Science and Vedic Wisdom

Modern neuroscience and Vedic traditions agree: nutrition is the cornerstone of cognitive health. Here are foods to fuel your brain:

Modern Science:

- **Omega-3 Fatty Acids**: Found in salmon and flaxseeds; crucial for brain cell structure.
- **Berries**: Packed with antioxidants to reduce oxidative stress.
- **Dark Chocolate**: Improves blood flow and focus with flavonoids.

Vedic Wisdom:

- **Ghee**: Nourishes the brain and enhances clarity.
- **Amla (Indian Gooseberry)**: A potent antioxidant for mental sharpness.
- **Turmeric**: Promotes neurogenesis through anti-**inflammatory properties.**

Combining these traditions offers a holistic approach to nourishing your mind.

Closing thoughts: Fueling a Limitless Mind

A limitless mind isn't born—it's cultivated. By mastering your mindset, aligning with your motivation, and employing effective learning methods, you can shatter mental barriers and achieve extraordinary cognitive performance. Remember: growth thrives on persistence, self-care, and the unrelenting belief in your ability to evolve.

11 HARNESSING TECHNOLOGY FOR HEALTH

"An ounce of prevention is worth a pound of cure"

— *Benjamin Franklin*

Biohacking has evolved far beyond taking supplements or fine-tuning your workout routine. In the pursuit of optimal health and performance, integrating cutting-edge technology is no longer a luxury—it has become essential for those striving to achieve greater personal limits. From wearable devices that monitor every facet of our health to therapies utilizing light, sound, and electricity for enhanced recovery, modern biohacking provides tools to optimize the body and mind with precision. With modern biosensors and wearable health monitors, you can take charge of your health like never before! These devices provide real-time insights into metrics like blood sugar, heart rate, and stress levels, empowering you to make proactive lifestyle adjustments. From optimizing workouts to managing chronic conditions, frequent monitoring helps you stay ahead and in control of your well-being.

In this chapter, we will delve into various technologies and devices designed to accelerate wellness, boost performance, and sharpen mental clarity, leading to a higher quality of life. Whether your goal is to improve physical health, optimize sleep, or enhance cognitive function, technology offers solutions that complement natural biohacking efforts.

Here are some popular therapeutic biohacking devices designed to optimize health and performance:

1. Red Light Therapy (Photobiomodulation)

ATP (Adenosine Triphosphate) is the cell's energy currency. ATP production using the normal food cycle involves multiple complex steps: ingestion, digestion, absorption, transport, cellular uptake, and respiration. This process is dependent on macronutrient breakdown and typically takes hours to generate substantial energy. In contrast, near-infrared (NIR) light therapy accelerates ATP production directly within mitochondria without requiring food digestion or absorption. Here's a step-by-step comparison:

Normal Food Cycle:
- Energy Source: Proteins, carbohydrates, and

fats.

- Timeframe: Hours (from ingestion to cellular respiration).
- ATP Production Pathway: Nutrients are metabolized through glycolysis, the citric acid cycle, and the electron transport chain (ETC).
- ATP yield is dependent on the complete metabolic breakdown of macronutrients.
- Efficiency: Energy generation can be delayed due to digestion, absorption inefficiencies, or nutrient availability.
- Oxidative stress and metabolic byproducts can accumulate, potentially leading to inefficiencies.

Near-Infrared (NIR) Light Therapy:

- **Energy Source:** Photons of light in the NIR spectrum (600–1100 nm).
- **Timeframe:** Immediate effect as photons are absorbed directly by tissues.
- **ATP Production Pathway**: NIR light penetrates the skin and is absorbed by mitochondrial chromophores (e.g., cytochrome c oxidase).
- This directly energizes the electron transport chain (ETC), bypassing the need for nutrient breakdown or transport.
- **Efficiency:** Faster ATP production due to the direct stimulation of mitochondrial activity.

- Improves efficiency by reducing oxidative stress and enhancing oxygen utilization.

NIR Light and Mitochondrial Function

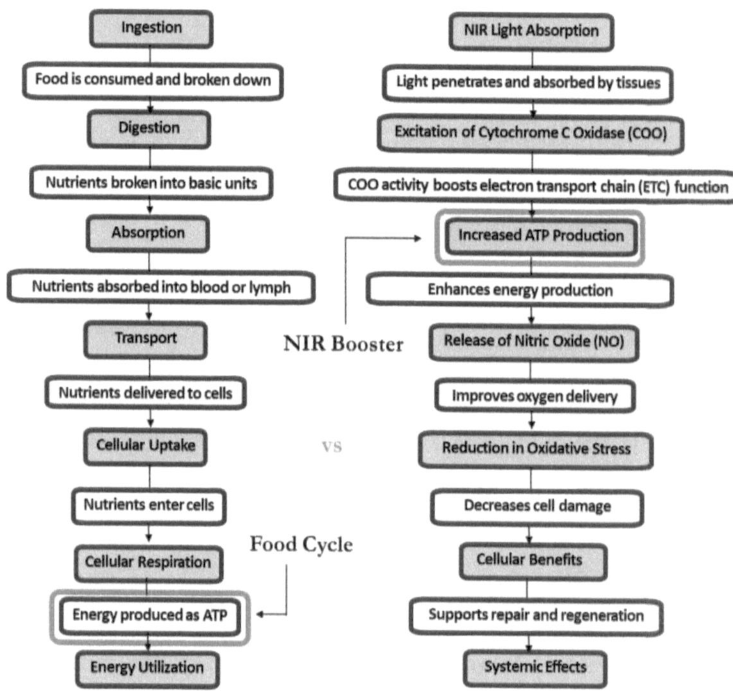

The primary source of near-infrared radiation (NIR) is the sun. Solar NIR makes up a significant portion of the sunlight reaching the Earth's surface. Getting NIR light from the sun early in the morning is tricky because the sun's spectrum at dawn is heavily skewed towards visible (400–700 nm) and blue wavelengths due to atmospheric scattering effects. The intensity of NIR, which is vital for certain health benefits, is relatively low during these hours.

To ensure consistent and adequate NIR exposure, especially in less sunny regions or during overcast days, devices like NIR lamps or panels are essential. These devices provide controlled and targeted doses of this beneficial wavelength, overcoming the variability and limitations of natural sunlight.

Red Light Therapy Devices

Red light therapy combines red and NIR light to accelerate repair, reduce inflammation, and improve skin health. Devices like Joovv Red Light Therapy Panels and PlatinumLED Biomax Panels deliver targeted doses of light, aiding recovery and improving energy levels.

Whether through natural sunlight or specialized devices, consistent red light therapy supports cellular health, vitality, and overall performance.

Key Systemic Effects of NIR Light:

1. **Improved Cellular Energy (ATP) Production**

   NIR light stimulates the mitochondria, the energy powerhouses of cells, by enhancing the activity of cytochrome c oxidase, a critical enzyme in the electron transport chain. This results in increased ATP production, providing energy for cellular repair and regeneration.

2. Enhanced Blood Circulation

NIR light promotes vasodilation by increasing the production of nitric oxide (NO), a molecule that relaxes blood vessels. This improves oxygen and nutrient delivery to tissues and facilitates the removal of metabolic waste.

3. Reduced Inflammation

By modulating inflammatory pathways, NIR light can decrease the production of pro-inflammatory cytokines and increase anti-inflammatory markers, leading to systemic anti-inflammatory effects.

4. Pain Relief

NIR light reduces pain signals by desensitizing nociceptors (pain receptors) and promoting the release of endorphins. These effects can be felt throughout the body, even if only specific areas are treated.

5. Immune System Modulation

NIR light can enhance immune cell activity, improving the body's ability to fight infections and heal wounds. It may also modulate autoimmune responses to reduce systemic inflammation.

6. Neuroprotective Benefits

When applied to the head, NIR light may cross the skull and enhance brain function by reducing oxidative stress, promoting neurogenesis (growth of new neurons), and improving brain metabolism. These effects can influence overall mental clarity and mood.

7. Systemic Detoxification

NIR light therapy can activate the lymphatic system, which aids in the removal of toxins and waste products from the body.

2. Wearable Technology – The Data You Need for Real-Time Health Tracking

Wearable technology has revolutionized health optimization by providing real-time insights into metrics such as heart rate and sleep cycles. These devices act as personal health assistants, offering feedback to help you make smarter decisions about your lifestyle, workouts, and recovery. Key wearables include:

- **Smartwatches & Fitness Trackers**: Devices like the Apple Watch and Garmin track heart rate, oxygen saturation (SpO2), and activity levels, delivering comprehensive data to fine-tune your health routine.
- **Continuous Glucose Monitors (CGMs)**: For biohackers focused on metabolic health, CGMs like Freestyle Libre and Dexcom provide real-time glucose tracking, enabling a better understanding of how food, exercise, and stress impact blood sugar.
- **Sleep Trackers**: Tools such as the Oura Ring

and WHOOP Strap offer insights into sleep quality, empowering you to optimize rest for recovery and mental clarity.

By leveraging the data provided by these devices, you can adjust behaviors to achieve optimal wellness.

3. Portable Diagnostic Devices – At-Home Testing for Precision Health

At-home diagnostic tools simplify taking charge of your health by offering the ability to test for nutrient deficiencies, track biomarkers, and monitor conditions without clinic visits.

- **Genetic and Microbiome Testing**: Companies like 23andMe and Viome analyze your genetics and microbiome, providing personalized insights to optimize diet, exercise, and overall health.
- **Blood Pressure Monitors & ECG Devices**: Devices such as Withings Blood Pressure Monitor and KardiaMobile enable cardiovascular health tracking, helping detect irregularities early and prompting proactive lifestyle adjustments.

These diagnostic tools empower biohackers to stay ahead of health challenges and personalize strategies for wellness.

4. Neurofeedback and Brain Stimulation – Optimizing Mental Performance

Neurofeedback and brain stimulation technologies help enhance cognitive function, mood, and mental clarity by directly interacting with brain activity.

- **Muse Headband**: Provides real-time brain-wave feedback during meditation, enabling deeper relaxation and focus.
- **Halo Neurostimulation**: Uses transcranial electrical stimulation to boost focus, learning, and cognitive performance.
- **tDCS Devices**: Tools like the Fisher Wallace Stimulator use mild electrical currents to treat anxiety or depression while improving cognitive function.

These devices allow you to "hack" your brain for improved learning, productivity, and emotional well-being.

5. Sleep Optimization – Enhancing Rest for Peak Performance

Optimizing sleep is critical for recovery, mental clarity, and well-being. Technology helps track and enhance sleep patterns for better rest.

- **Smart Sleep Trackers**: Products like the Eight Sleep Pod Pro and Oura Ring monitor temperature, heart rate, and deep sleep, ensuring an ideal sleep environment.
- **Sound Therapy & White Noise**: Devices such as LectroFan or apps offering binaural

beats help reduce distractions and promote relaxation.

- **Blue Light-Blocking Tools**: Glasses or smart lighting systems like Philips Hue help maintain natural circadian rhythms by reducing exposure to artificial blue light.

By leveraging these tools, you can optimize sleep, laying the foundation for improved health and performance.

6. Infrared Saunas and Heat Therapy – Detoxification and Circulation Boost

Infrared saunas use infrared light to heat the body directly, promoting deep tissue detoxification, relaxation, and enhanced circulation.

- **Popular Devices**: Sunlighten Infrared Saunas and HigherDOSE Sauna Blankets.
- **Combination with Cold Therapy**: Pairing heat therapy with cold treatments like ice baths can further enhance recovery and reduce inflammation.

7. Air and Water Quality Enhancers – Creating a Healthy Environment

Clean air and water are critical for health. Technology can improve the quality of your living environment.

- **Air Purifiers**: Devices such as Molekule or Dyson Purifiers remove allergens and pollutants.
- **Water Filters**: Systems like Berkey Filters or

"He who has
health has hope
and he who has
hope has
everything."
— Arabian Proverb

Reverse Osmosis Units provide clean, contaminant-free water.

Optimizing your environment is as important as optimizing your body.

8. Virtual Reality (VR) for Wellness – Immersive Stress Reduction

VR platforms such as TRIPP and RELAXVR offer immersive experiences for guided meditation, nature immersion, and stress reduction, providing innovative ways to enhance mental health.

9. Sound Therapy – Enhancing Focus and Sleep

Sound therapy tools can improve focus, relaxation, and sleep through various frequencies and soundscapes.

- **White Noise Machines**: Devices like Lectro-Fan mask environmental noise for better concentration or sleep.
- **Binaural Beats Apps**: Tools like Brain.fm promote relaxation and focus through auditory stimulation.

Closing Thoughts:

Biohacking leverages advanced tools like heart rate monitors, continuous glucose monitors (CGMs), and sleep trackers to revolutionize health optimization. By tracking key metrics—resting heart rate (60–100 bpm; 40–60 bpm for athletes), active heart rate (120–160 bpm during exercise), oxygen saturation (95–100%

SpO2), steps (10,000/day), and calories burned—we gain insights to enhance fitness and activity levels.

CGMs empower personalized nutrition, monitoring fasting glucose (70–99 mg/dL for non-diabetics) and postprandial levels (<140 mg/dL). Sleep trackers optimize rest by ensuring 7–9 hours of total sleep, with 10–25% deep sleep and 20–25% REM sleep, achieving an ideal score (85+).

For older adults, health tracking ensures safety, enhances chronic disease management, and supports emotional and cognitive health, enabling them to age gracefully. For younger generations, it fosters healthy habits, boosts academic and athletic performance, and promotes mental resilience, setting the stage for a lifetime of wellness.

From monitoring vital signs to empowering mental health, from preventive care to personalized insights, these advancements redefine what's possible for both present and future health. With real-time data, proactive adjustments, and professional collaboration, we can not only address today's health challenges but also build a healthier tomorrow.

Health tracking is more than a tool—it's a lifelong ally in achieving well-being, empowering us to live healthier, happier, and more fulfilling lives.

12 THE MOVEMENT MATRIX

"Movement is medicine"

—Anonymous

The human body is a marvel of engineering, designed for dynamic movement and motion. With over 360 joints and 700 skeletal muscles, every inch of our anatomy is primed to support an active lifestyle—not to endure the stagnation of prolonged sitting. Motion isn't just a preference; it's a necessity.

Did you know? During exercise, your muscles can absorb glucose directly from the bloodstream without needing insulin!

Exercise is a powerful biohack that elevates physical performance, mental clarity, and overall well-being. Contrary to the flashy world of billionaires, you don't need expensive tools or endless time to optimize your workouts. The only bad workout is the one you didn't do.

Movement has a profound impact on glucose regulation in the body, acting as a natural sink for glucose. When muscles contract during physical activity, they require energy to perform work. This energy is primarily derived from glucose and fatty acids stored in the body. Every squat, step, and stretch make your muscles a natural sugar sink. Here's how it works:

How Muscles Soak Up Glucose During Movement

1. **Insulin-Independent Glucose Uptake**: Unlike rest, during exercise, muscles can absorb glucose without the need for insulin. Muscle contractions stimulate glucose transporter type 4 (GLUT4) to move to the cell surface, where it facilitates glucose entry into muscle cells.

2. **Increased Blood Flow**: Movement enhances blood flow to active muscles, delivering more glucose and oxygen to fuel activity.

3. **Depletion of Glycogen Stores**: During exercise, muscles use stored glycogen (a glucose polymer) as an energy source. This depletion signals the body to replenish these stores by pulling more glucose from the bloodstream post-exercise.

4. **Improved Insulin Sensitivity**: Regular movement increases insulin sensitivity, meaning cells become

more efficient at using glucose even after the activity ends.

Why Movement Acts as a Glucose Sink

Muscles are the largest glucose storage site in the body. They are glucose sponges—move them, and they clean the system. During movement:

- **Glucose Demand Rises**: Active muscles use glucose at a much higher rate than at rest, effectively lowering blood sugar levels.
- **Post-Exercise Recovery**: After movement, muscles act like sponges, soaking up glucose to replenish glycogen stores, keeping blood sugar levels balanced.

Health Benefits of This Process

1. **Blood Sugar Control**: Regular movement helps prevent spikes in blood sugar levels and reduces the risk of type 2 diabetes.

2. **Weight Management**: By utilizing glucose effectively, movement helps in burning calories and managing body weight.

3. **Improved Metabolic Health**: Exercise-induced

glucose uptake supports overall metabolic function, reducing the risk of insulin resistance and associated chronic conditions.

Even simple movements, like walking after meals, can significantly enhance glucose uptake by muscles, making movement one of the most effective tools for maintaining healthy blood sugar levels. Here is how you can start:

Define Your Why and Set Measurable Goals

Clarifying your purpose helps tailor your routine. Use specific metrics to measure success:

Goal: Strength and Power

- Metric: Measure increases in max lifts (e.g., deadlift, squat, bench press).
- Example: Aim for a 10% increase in your one-rep max every 8 weeks.

Goal: Endurance

- Metric: Improve VO_2 max (maximum oxygen uptake during exercise). Your body needs oxygen to produce energy for exercise. VO_2 max measures how efficiently your body can use that oxygen.
- Example: Target a VO_2 max increase from 35 to 40 mL/kg/min in 3 months.

"Sweat is just fat crying. Move until the tears stop."

– Jillian Michaels

Goal: Mental Clarity and Focus

- Metric: Track mood and energy levels post-workout using a journal or app.

Here's how to customize your weekly workout routine:

1. Warm-Up: Prime Your Body for Optimal Performance

An effective warm-up enhances performance and minimizes injury risk.

- **Dynamic Stretching**: Incorporate movements like lunges or arm circles for 5–10 minutes to improve range of motion.
- **Heart Rate Activation**: Gradually elevate your heart rate to 50–60% of your max (calculated as 220 minus your age).
- **VO₂ Max Training Prep**: For VO_2 max optimization, start with 5 minutes of moderate jogging or cycling to prepare for intervals.

2. Smart Workouts: Boost Results with Efficiency

Time-efficient exercises can yield incredible gains:

High-Intensity Interval Training (HIIT)

- Protocol: 30 seconds of intense effort (85–95% of max heart rate), followed by 1–2 minutes of active recovery.

- Goal: Complete 4–6 cycles per session.
- Metric: Track performance by improving average distance covered or calories burned during intervals.

Resistance Training

- Focus: Compound movements (e.g., squats, deadlifts) to engage multiple muscle groups.
- Metric: Monitor progression by increasing weight, reps, or sets weekly.

Endurance and VO$_2$ Max

Example: Perform tempo runs at 75–85% of max heart rate for 20–30 minutes.

3. Use Wearables to Track Progress

Affordable fitness trackers and apps can monitor essential metrics:

- **VO$_2$ Max**: Some devices estimate your VO$_2$ max based on heart rate and activity data.
- **Heart Rate Zones**: Stay within optimal ranges for endurance (60–80%) or HIIT (80–95%).
- **Step Count**: Aim for 8,000–10,000 daily steps to stay active outside workouts.

4. Recovery: The Unsung Hero of Fitness

Recovery optimizes performance and prevents burnout:

Cold Exposure: Try 3–5 minutes of cold showers or ice baths post-exercise.

- Metric: Measure reduced muscle soreness or faster heart rate recovery time.
- **Heart Rate Variability (HRV)**: Use apps or wearables to track HRV—a higher score indicates better recovery.
- **Active Recovery**: Dedicate 1–2 days a week to low-intensity activities like yoga or walking.

5. Nutrition for Exercise Success

Fuel your workouts and recovery with the right foods:

Pre-Workout

- Goal: Stabilize energy levels.
- Example: Eat a banana with peanut butter or oatmeal 1–2 hours before exercising.

Post-Workout

- Goal: Muscle repair and glycogen replenishment.
- Example: Consume 20–30g of protein and 40–60g of carbs, like a smoothie with protein powder, berries, and spinach.
- **Hydration:** Monitor hydration by checking urine color (clear to light yellow indicates adequate hydration).

6. Hack Your Environment

Create a space that enhances your workout experience:

- **Temperature Control**: Keep the room between 60–70°F for optimal performance.
- **Noise and Focus**: Use noise-canceling headphones with playlists tuned to your workout goals (e.g., high-energy beats for HIIT).

7. Measure and Improve VO₂ Max

VO$_2$ max is a vital metric for cardiovascular fitness and endurance. Here's how to enhance it:

Interval Training

- Protocol: Perform 4-minute intervals at 85–90% of your max heart rate, followed by 3-minute recovery periods.
- Metric: Reassess VO$_2$ max every 6–8 weeks using wearables or fitness tests.

Consistency

Goal: Train at least 3 times per week, including 1–2 sessions focused on aerobic intensity.

8. Incorporate Daily Movement

Small, consistent actions keep you active throughout the day:

- **Break the Sedentary Cycle**: Set a timer to stand or stretch every hour.

Sample Weekly Workout Routine

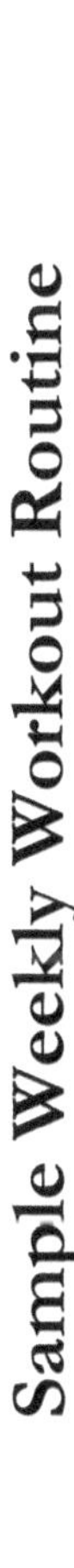

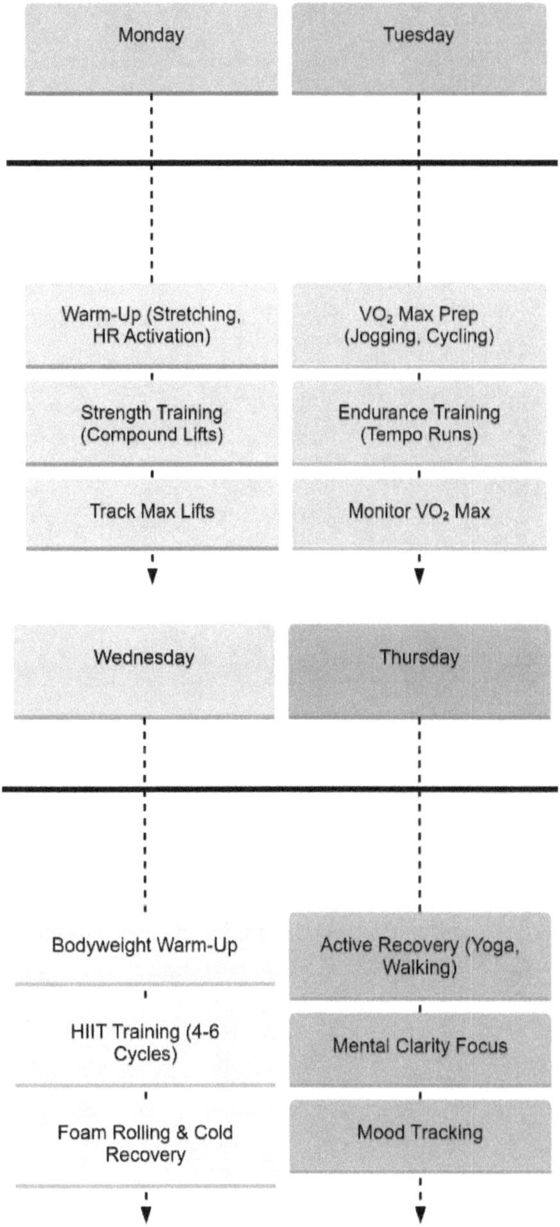
Monday
Tuesday
Warm-Up (Stretching, HR Activation)
VO₂ Max Prep (Jogging, Cycling)
Strength Training (Compound Lifts)
Endurance Training (Tempo Runs)
Track Max Lifts
Monitor VO₂ Max
Wednesday
Thursday
Bodyweight Warm-Up
Active Recovery (Yoga, Walking)
HIIT Training (4-6 Cycles)
Mental Clarity Focus
Foam Rolling & Cold Recovery
Mood Tracking

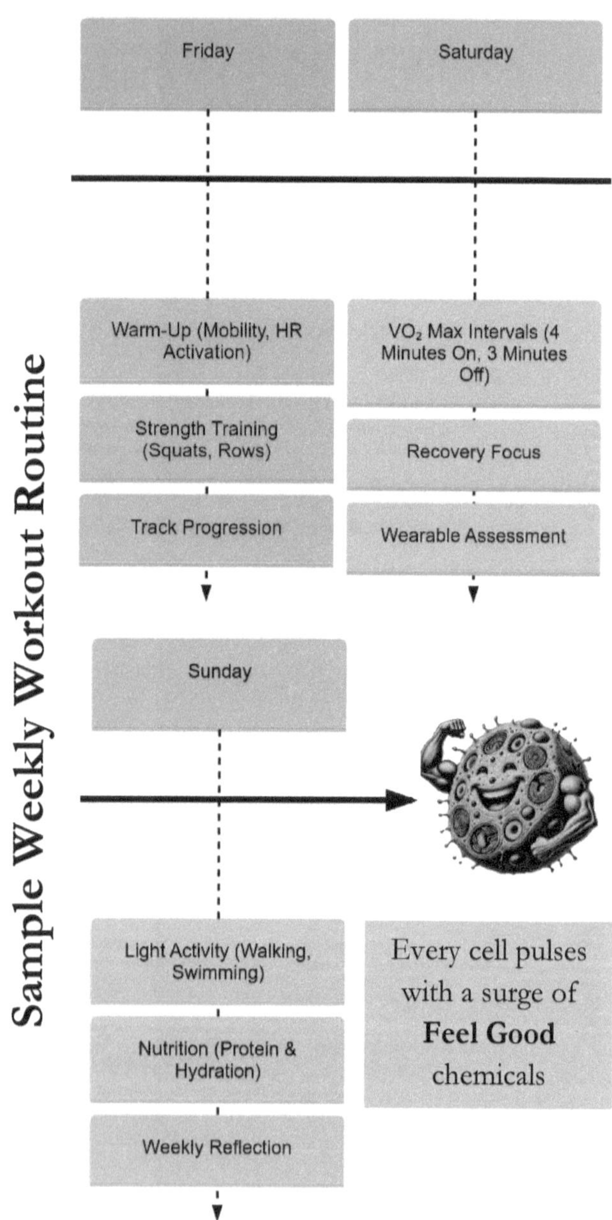

Sample Weekly Workout Routine
Friday
Saturday
Warm-Up (Mobility, HR Activation)
VO₂ Max Intervals (4 Minutes On, 3 Minutes Off)
Strength Training (Squats, Rows)
Recovery Focus
Track Progression
Wearable Assessment
Sunday
Light Activity (Walking, Swimming)
Nutrition (Protein & Hydration)
Weekly Reflection
Every cell pulses with a surge of Feel Good chemicals

- **Walking Meetings**: Substitute sitting with walking during discussions.
- **Metrics**: Track daily movement with step counters or accelerometers.

By combining biohacking principles with actionable metrics, you can elevate your fitness routine for better performance, recovery, and health—without a billionaire budget.

Make Movement a Lifestyle

Feeling tired and out of focus? You're not alone—but there's a simple solution, and it doesn't come in a coffee cup.

Research shows that even short bursts of physical activity, known as "acute exercise," can spark a cascade of brain-enhancing chemicals.

Neurotransmitters like dopamine, GABA, and acetylcholine flood your system, boosting communication between brain cells. At the same time, Brain-Derived Neurotrophic Factor (BDNF) strengthens neural connections, improving memory and focus.

The best part? You don't need hours at the gym to reap these benefits. A quick walk, desk stretches, or a few squats can clear mental fog, reduce stress, and recharge your mind. And if you time your movement before or during demanding tasks, the benefits multiply.

High-intensity activities amplify results, but even moderate movement can transform a sluggish brain into a powerhouse of clarity.

So, the next time you feel stuck, step away, move, and let your mind thrive. Start small. Start now. Your brain—and your productivity—will thank you.

Here's a curated list of biohacks designed to integrate movement seamlessly into your day:

1. After Meals: Take a Walk
- Action: Walk for 10 minutes post-meal.
- Benefit: Aids digestion, stabilizes blood sugar, and boosts circulation.

2. Brushing Your Teeth: Add Squats
- Action: Perform bodyweight squats or calf raises while brushing.
- Benefit: Activates muscles and improves balance in just 2 minutes.

3. During Phone Calls: Pace or Stretch
- Action: Walk around or do standing stretches while on the phone.
- Benefit: Combines activity with productivity, reducing sedentary time.

4. Watching TV: Use Commercial Breaks
- Action: Stretch or do light yoga poses during commercials.
- Benefit: Improves flexibility and prevents prolonged sitting.

5. Before Bed: Gentle Yoga

- Action: Practice a short yoga routine or light stretches.
- Benefit: Relaxes muscles and enhances sleep quality.

6. Upon Waking: Morning Flow

- Action: Start your day with 5 minutes of stretches, lunges, or spinal twists.
- Benefit: Boosts circulation and prepares your body for the day ahead.

7. Waiting in Line: Balance Work

- Action: Stand on one leg or shift weight side-to-side.
- Benefit: Engages stabilizing muscles and improves core strength.

8. At Your Desk: Desk Yoga

- Action: Perform seated stretches or simple desk yoga poses.
- Benefit: Relieves tension and increases blood flow during work hours.

9. Lunch Breaks: Step Outside

- Action: Take a walk outdoors during lunch.
- Benefit: Refreshes the mind, provides sunlight, and promotes movement.

10. Cooking: Step and Strengthen

- Action: Use a sturdy surface for step-ups or incline push-ups while waiting.
- Benefit: Adds functional strength exercises to daily chores.

11. After Meetings: Reset with Movement

- Action: Take a 5-minute dance break or do

light stretches.

- Benefit: Resets energy and focus after sitting through long meetings.

12. Commuting: Park Farther Away

- Action: Park farther from your destination or exit public transport a stop early.
- Benefit: Increases daily step count effortlessly.

13. Brewing Coffee: Add Planks

- Action: Hold a plank or do counter push-ups while your coffee brews.
- Benefit: Builds core strength and upper body endurance.

14. After Work: Decompress with Exercise

- Action: Go for a brisk walk or hit the gym.
- Benefit: Reduces stress and boosts endorphin levels.

15. Feeling Sluggish: Stretch and Breathe

- Action: Perform a quick stretch routine paired with deep breathing.
- Benefit: Re-energizes and sharpens mental focus.

16. Playtime: Join the Kids

- Action: Engage in active play with children.
- Benefit: Increases movement while fostering bonding and fun.

17. Hourly Sitting Breaks: Stand and Stretch

- Action: Set a timer to stand and stretch every hour.
- Benefit: Counteracts the negative effects of prolonged sitting.

18. Folding Laundry: Add Lunges

- Action: Incorporate reverse lunges or side lunges between folding tasks.
- Benefit: Turns a chore into a strength-training opportunity.

19. Grocery Shopping: Engage Your Core

- Action: Walk with a slight core contraction while pushing the cart.
- Benefit: Strengthens stability muscles and improves posture.

20. Before Eating: Activate with Squats

- Action: Do 10 air squats or light jumping jacks before meals.
- Benefit: Primes your metabolism and stimulates circulation.

Closing Thoughts: Make Exercise Non-Negotiable

By embedding physical activity into the rhythm of your day, you're not just improving your body, you're enhancing your mind, elevating your mood, and boosting your focus. And as these small habits take root, you'll find that being active becomes second nature, rather than a chore. The secret is consistency, not perfection. Make exercise your daily priority, and you'll find yourself enjoying a more energized, balanced, and healthier lifestyle—one small step at a time.

13 BIO-CHIC

" Style isn't just what you wear; it's how you care—for yourself and the planet. "

—Anonymous

Living bio-chic means embodying a lifestyle that is equal parts stylish, health-conscious, and sustainable. It's about making intentional choices that prioritize personal well-being, environmental stewardship, and a sense of refined elegance. From the clothes you wear to the products you use, every detail reflects a commitment to thriving in harmony with the world around you.

Endocrine Disruptors: The Hidden Threat

In our pursuit of beauty and convenience, we often overlook the invisible dangers lurking in everyday products. Endocrine disruptors, harmful chemicals that interfere with the body's hormonal systems, are commonly found in items we use daily:

The Culprits

1. **Detergents & Fabric Softeners**: Contain phthalates and triclosan, which disrupt reproductive hormones.
2. **Perfumes & Fragrances**: Synthetic musks mimic estrogen, potentially causing developmental issues.
3. **Cosmetics**: Parabens, BHA, and BHT contribute to hormonal imbalances and cancer risks.
4. **Shampoos & Conditioners**: Sulfates and parabens impact fertility and overall hormone balance.
5. **Clothing & Fabrics**: BPA, formaldehyde, and perfluorochemicals (PFCs) are endocrine disruptors in synthetic materials.
6. **Cleaners & Pesticides**: Glyphosate and triclosan interfere with thyroid and reproductive hormones.

Bio-Chic Alternatives

- Opt for organic fabrics like cotton, hemp, or linen.
- Use natural detergents and fragrance-free products.
- Transition to mineral-based sunscreens and non-toxic skincare products.

By making these choices, you shield your body from harmful toxins while fostering a cleaner planet.

"When you have a choice, choose wisely"

–Anonymous

The Bio-Chic Checklist: Metrics for a Holistic Lifestyle

Living bio-chic is about measurable progress. Here's how to embrace this lifestyle:

1. **Clothing**
   - **Natural Fabrics**: Aim for 70% of your wardrobe to be made from organic, eco-friendly materials.
   - **Sustainable Brands**: Commit to buying 80% of your clothing from ethical or environmentally-conscious brands.
   - **Vintage Finds**: Make 30% of your wardrobe secondhand or vintage.

2. **Personal Care**
   - **Toxin-Free Beauty**: Replace 80% of products with organic, non-toxic options free from parabens and phthalates.
   - **DIY Skincare**: Incorporate two DIY skincare recipes into your routine monthly.
   - **Eco-Friendly Tools**: Use bamboo toothbrushes, reusable cotton pads, and natural loofahs for 100% of your beauty regimen.

3. **Daily Habits**
   - **Mindful Self-Care**: Dedicate 30 minutes daily to rituals like meditation, yoga, or dry brushing.
   - **Balanced Living**: Get 7–9 hours of sleep,

consume five servings of vegetables, and exercise 3–5 times weekly.

- **Gratitude Journaling**: End each day reflecting on three things you're thankful for.

4. **Conscious Shopping**
   - **Ethical Purchases**: Ensure 80% of your home goods, groceries, and clothing are sustainable and cruelty-free.
   - **Reusable Items**: Use reusable bags and containers 100% of the time.
   - **Locally Sourced Foods**: Buy at least 50% of your groceries from local farmers or organic markets.

A Day in the Life of a Bio-Chic

Balancing mind, body, and soul with a fusion of science, wellness, and style.

Morning: Energizing the Mind and Body

- Wake up to the soft sounds of nature, embracing gratitude for a new day. Begin with a glass of warm water infused with lemon or tulsi (holy basil) to cleanse and hydrate.
- Kick off the day with gentle yoga or tai chi to energize and center yourself, followed by pranayama or box breathing to clear the mind.
- Enjoy a wholesome breakfast rooted in Asian

flavors: a bowl of congee with ginger and scallions, poached eggs, or dosa with a side of chutney and steamed veggies.

- Dress in breathable, elegant clothing, blending traditional fabrics like cotton or silk with modern styles for a functional yet fashionable look.
- Dive into work with mindful focus and purpose.

Afternoon: Balanced Nourishment

- Relish a balanced lunch featuring staples: a nourishing miso soup, stir-fried vegetables with tofu, or a wholesome sushi platter. Complement this with a light walk to refresh your mind and stay active.
- Take quick movement breaks, perhaps practicing a few minutes of qigong or light stretches to sustain focus and prevent fatigue.
- Recharge with a snack: a handful of roasted nuts, matcha tea, or fresh fruit like guava, lychee, or mango for a natural energy boost.
- Tackle the latter half of the day with renewed vigor, keeping your workspace uncluttered to promote mental clarity.

Evening: Relax, Reflect, and Recharge

- As the sun sets, enjoy a tranquil dinner such as steamed fish with bok choy, kimchi, and brown rice, incorporating spices like turmeric and cumin for added health benefits.

- Decompress with a soothing bath infused with jasmine or sandalwood essential oils, followed by a calming skincare ritual.
- Reflect on the day with journaling or share meaningful conversations with family over a pot of herbal tea like chamomile or chrysanthemum.
- Wind down by reading a book on wellness, watching an uplifting Korean drama, or meditating. Prepare for restful sleep with light stretches and setting intentions for tomorrow.

A Decade of Bio-Chic Living: A Glimpse into Your Radiant Future

Imagine this: a decade from now, you're striding into your golden years—not limping, not shuffling, but walking tall with the vitality of someone half your age. Bio-Chic living, the art of balancing wellness, science, and style, isn't just a daily ritual; it's your passport to aging gracefully, energetically, and joyfully.

Your mornings are vibrant, fueled by years of mindful choices. Decades of nourishing breakfasts, yoga flows, and gratitude practices have gifted you a body that feels agile and a mind that feels sharp. Gone are the days of groaning joints and sluggish starts; instead, you rise with purpose, your energy as boundless as the sun.

Your gut, once a silent participant, now works as your second brain. It hums with health, thanks to your dedication to probiotics, fermented foods, and fiber-packed meals. You no longer feel the dreaded post-meal fog. Instead, your digestion is a symphony of efficiency, fueling a life of clarity and vigor.

As you glance in the mirror, you notice the glow. Not just skin-deep but radiating from within. Years of hydration, nutrient-rich foods, and stress management have sculpted a visage that speaks of health, not haste. The wrinkles that do exist? They're badges of laughter, not worry.

Your relationships have deepened, built on the foundation of emotional resilience and mindfulness cultivated over the years. Bio-Chic living hasn't just made you healthier—it's made you present. The family dinners, shared walks, and heart-to-heart conversations have filled your life with warmth, love, and connection.

When others your age lament about aches, chronic illnesses, and a lack of energy, you smile knowingly. The investments you made in your health—a decade of balanced meals, regular movement, and a commitment to rest—have paid dividends. Your evenings are still filled with passion projects, whether it's gardening, dancing, or exploring a new skill.

In the end, Bio-Chic living is not about adding years to

your life; it's about adding life to your years. It's about thriving, not merely surviving. So here's to the next decade of chic, intentional living—because growing older isn't about slowing down; it's about embracing every moment with the vibrancy of someone who chose to live well.

Closing Thoughts: Living Bio-Chic

The bio-chic lifestyle is more than a trend—it's a movement toward intentional, sustainable, and health-focused living. It's about looking and feeling your best while protecting the planet and creating a life that radiates elegance and well-being.

Every choice you make, from the products you use to the habits you cultivate, shapes your journey to a more vibrant, balanced, and fulfilled life. Step into the bio-chic world and watch your life transform.

14 BURNOUT TO BRILLIANCE CHECKLIST

" It's not the load that breaks you, it's the way

you carry it"

— Lou Holtz

Life, at its core, is a tapestry of contradictions—a paradox where seemingly opposing forces coexist, shaping our existence and growth. These paradoxes are not flaws in the design of life but its essential features, teaching us profound lessons about balance, meaning, and transformation. Here's a reflection on the paradox of life:

1.   To Gain, We Must Lose

Life teaches us that growth often comes at the cost of letting go. We must lose comfort to gain wisdom, surrender stability to embrace adventure, and shed old identities to uncover our true selves. Loss is not the end; it is the clearing ground for renewal.

2. Strength Lies in Vulnerability

True strength is not the absence of weakness but the courage to embrace it. By being vulnerable, we forge deeper connections, foster trust, and discover resilience. It is in admitting what we lack that we gain the power to grow.

3. Freedom Through Discipline

While freedom seems to oppose structure, it is through discipline that we unlock true liberation. By committing to a practice, a purpose, or a vision, we create the space to explore, innovate, and transcend limitations.

4. Joy Springs from Sorrow

The sweetness of joy is understood only through the bitterness of sorrow. Life's happiest moments gain their depth and meaning because they are framed by challenges and loss. Without sorrow, joy would be hollow, a mere fleeting sensation.

5. The More We Know, the Less We Understand

Knowledge expands our horizons but also reveals the vastness of the unknown. Each answer uncovers deeper questions, reminding us of the infinite complexity of existence. True wisdom lies in embracing our ignorance and remaining curious.

6. Control Is Found in Letting Go

The harder we cling to control, the more elusive it becomes. Life flows most freely when we surrender to its natural rhythms, trusting the process and allowing things to unfold in their own time. Letting go is not giving up; it's making space for possibilities.

7. Life Is Both Finite and Infinite

While our physical existence is bound by time, the impact of our actions, ideas, and relationships extends far beyond our mortal frame. We live in the moment but echo through eternity, embodying the paradox of permanence and impermanence.

8. Individuality and Interconnectedness

We strive to define ourselves as unique individuals, yet our existence is deeply intertwined with others. Our individuality gains meaning through relationships, and our collective humanity is enriched by diversity.

The paradox of life challenges us to accept that contradictions are not to be resolved but embraced. They are the essence of what makes life dynamic, beautiful, and profoundly meaningful. By living within these tensions, we find not answers but deeper questions—and in them, the richness of the human experience.

So, the next time you find yourself at the edge of exhaustion, take a step back. Embrace the paradox. Recognize that burnout may just be the precursor to brilliance, and in the dance between these two seemingly opposing forces, you might discover the most powerful version of yourself. It's not about avoiding burnout—it's about learning how to transform it, how to turn that exhaustion into fuel for the brilliance waiting to emerge.

Switching from burnout to brilliance requires more than rest; it demands a holistic, creative approach to recharging mind, body, and soul. True rejuvenation lies in breaking free from the endless cycle of depletion and rediscovering the spark that fuels your unique brilliance. It's about leaning into practices that nourish, inspire, and align you with your deepest purpose.

As the proverb goes, *"All work and no play makes Jack a dull boy."* Burnout often stems from neglecting the balance that play, creativity, and self-expression bring to life. Imagine a potter who spends years crafting the same type of vase over and over to meet demand, slowly losing the joy that drew them to the wheel in the first place. One day, they decide to break the routine and sculpt a wild, abstract piece that defies all convention. Though it doesn't serve their business directly, the act of creating something uniquely their own reignites their passion. They rediscover the artistry behind their craft, which fuels not only their work but their spirit.

Similarly, burnout often arises from suppressing your

untold story—your creative energy, passions, or authentic voice. As Maya Angelou eloquently said, *"There is no greater agony than bearing an untold story inside you."* When you allow that story to unfold, whether through innovation, personal projects, or introspection, you transition from mere survival to thriving. This expression becomes the bridge to brilliance, reigniting purpose and bringing every aspect of your life into alignment.

The journey from burnout to brilliance is not linear, but it is deeply transformative. Like the potter who rewrote the narrative of their craft, it calls for courage, self-awareness, and a willingness to explore what truly lights you up. By doing so, you not only give voice to the story within you but let it resonate powerfully with the world, illuminating your unique brilliance.

Here are some steps to guide you through this transformation:

1. Declutter Your Mind: The Brainstorm Break

- **How to Do It**: Take 10 minutes to jot down all the thoughts swirling in your mind—no structure, no filters, just free writing. This "brainstorm break" helps externalize the mental clutter, allowing you to step back and reset.
- **Why It Works**: Externalizing thoughts reduces mental load, giving your brain a chance to breathe and refocus.

"The secret to getting ahead is getting started."
– Mark Twain

2. Curate Your Energy: The Power Playlist

- **How to Do It**: Create a playlist with songs that elevate your energy or bring you peace. Whether it's empowering beats or relaxing tunes, use music to set the tone for your day.
- **Why It Works**: Music has a powerful impact on the brain, influencing mood, focus, and creativity, shifting you from a state of burnout to a state of brilliance.

3. Micro-Pause: The 5-Minute Zen

- **How to Do It**: Set an alarm for every hour, signaling a 5-minute "micro-pause." During this time, you can do something simple yet restorative—like breathing exercises, stretching, or staring out the window.
- **Why It Works**: Small, frequent breaks prevent mental exhaustion and help maintain focus, allowing you to regain energy and creativity throughout the day.

4. The Power of "No": The Boundary Challenge

- **How to Do It**: For the next 48 hours, say "no" to anything that drains your energy without guilt. Whether it's an unnecessary meeting, a task you can delegate, or a social commitment, protect your energy fiercely.
- **Why It Works**: Learning to say "no" helps you regain control over your time and energy, preventing further burnout while making space for

activities that light you up.

5. Nature Connection: The Forest Bath

- **How to Do It**: If possible, spend 15-30 minutes in nature—whether it's a walk through the park or sitting in your garden. Immerse yourself in the sights, sounds, and smells of the natural world.
- **Why It Works**: Nature has been scientifically shown to reduce stress, lower cortisol levels, and boost mood. This "nature reset" allows your body and mind to refresh and reset.

6. Creativity Unleashed: The Unusual Hobby

- **How to Do It**: Try a new creative hobby that excites you but isn't tied to productivity—pottery, painting, or even cooking a new recipe. Allow yourself to enjoy the process, not the outcome.
- **Why It Works**: Engaging in non-goal-oriented creative activities triggers the brain's reward system, lowering stress and reigniting inspiration.

7. Reframe Your Purpose: The "Why" Exercise

- **How to Do It**: Take 20 minutes to reflect on why you do what you do—whether it's your work, a personal project, or a passion. Write down your "big why" and revisit it daily.
- **Why It Works**: Reconnecting with your core

purpose reignites passion and drives, transforming feelings of burnout into a renewed
sense of meaning.

8. Sleep Reboot: The Restorative Night

- **How to Do It**: Commit to a week of sleep hygiene—consistent bedtime, no screens 30
minutes before sleep, and a calming pre-sleep
routine (like journaling or reading a book).
- **Why It Works**: Quality sleep is essential for
cognitive function, emotional balance, and
overall vitality, giving your mind the rest it
needs to perform at its best.

9. Gratitude Shift: The Magic 3

- **How to Do It**: Start and end your day by writing down three things you're grateful for. These
could be as simple as a good cup of coffee or
as profound as meaningful relationships.
- **Why It Works**: Gratitude rewires your brain to
focus on the positive, shifting your perspective
from burnout to brilliance by fostering feelings
of abundance.

10. Movement Breaks: The Mind-Body Reset

- **How to Do It**: During your day, integrate
small but impactful movements—like a 5-mi-
nute dance party, a short walk, or even a quick
stretch. These moments help to break up long
hours of sitting or mental strain.

- **Why It Works**: Physical activity triggers endorphins, boosts mood, and improves circulation, which helps to reset your body and mind.

11. Visualization: The Future Self

- **How to Do It**: Spend 5-10 minutes visualizing your ideal self, life, or next big achievement. Imagine how you feel, what you're doing, and who you're with.
- **Why It Works**: Visualization strengthens neural pathways related to success and confidence, shifting you into a positive and empowered mindset.

12. Social Detox: The Digital Declutter

- **How to Do It**: Disconnect from social media for a day (or more) to clear your mental space. Instead, focus on engaging in meaningful real-life interactions or simply being present with yourself.
- **Why It Works**: Digital detoxes reduce information overload and social comparison, helping you feel more connected to yourself and others.

13. The Power of Play: The Fun Break

- **How to Do It**: Allow yourself a "play" session—whether it's a spontaneous game, creative project, or playful interaction with loved ones.

- **Why It Works**: Play sparks joy, creativity, and stress relief, fostering a sense of freedom and flow that counteracts burnout.

14. Laughter Break: The Mood Lift

- **How to Do It**: Watch a funny video, listen to a comedy podcast, or spend time with someone who makes you laugh.
- **Why It Works**: Laughter increases endorphins and reduces cortisol, shifting you from burnout to a state of joy and clarity.

15. Mindful Eating: The Conscious Plate

- **How to Do It**: Instead of eating on autopilot, take time to truly savor every bite. Focus on texture, taste, and the nourishing qualities of your food.
- **Why It Works**: Mindful eating promotes digestion, reduces stress, and helps you reconnect with your body's needs.

16. Movement Meditation: The Flow State

- **How to Do It**: Practice **walking meditation** or **tai chi**, where the movement is synchronized with your breath, calming the mind while releasing physical tension.
- **Why It Works**: This type of mindful movement helps you reconnect with your body, balance energy, and focus attention, promoting a calm yet alert state.

17. Self-Compassion: The Kindness Habit

- **How to Do It**: Treat yourself with the same kindness and understanding you would offer a close friend. Whenever you feel burnout creeping in, remind yourself: "I am doing the best I can."
- **Why It Works**: Self-compassion reduces stress and enhances emotional resilience, helping you move from burnout to brilliance.

18. Affirmation Activation: The Empowerment Script

- **How to Do It**: Create an empowering affirmation that speaks to your current goals, energy, or mindset. Say it aloud or write it down daily.
- **Why It Works**: Affirmations reshape your mental landscape, encouraging self-belief and positive action.

19. Breathing Reset: The 4-7-8 Technique

- **How to Do It**: Try the 4-7-8 breathing **technique**: inhale for 4 seconds, hold for 7, and exhale for 8. Repeat 3-5 times.
- **Why It Works**: This technique activates the parasympathetic nervous system, reducing stress and promoting a sense of calm.

20. Celebrate Small Wins: The Gratitude Shout-Out

- **How to Do It**: Take time to celebrate even the

smallest accomplishments—completing a task, making progress, or simply surviving the day.

- **Why It Works**: Celebrating small wins fuels motivation, boosts mood, and helps you maintain momentum.

Closing Thoughts

Burnout is a powerful reminder of the consequences of neglecting our basic human needs, as highlighted by Michael Gungor's quote, *"Burnout is what happens when you try to avoid being human for too long."* In our relentless pursuit of perfection, productivity, and meeting external expectations, we often push ourselves beyond our limits, disregarding the essential human qualities of rest, connection, and self-compassion. This imbalance leads to physical, mental, and emotional exhaustion, ultimately affecting our ability to function effectively. The key to avoiding burnout lies in recognizing our vulnerability and embracing our humanity. Similarly, the quote *"You can't pour from an empty cup"* emphasizes the vital importance of self-care. To be able to give to others or perform at our best, we must first nourish and replenish ourselves. Prioritizing self-care ensures we maintain the energy, clarity, and resilience needed to face life's challenges with grace and effectiveness.

CLOSING NOTE: A HEARTFELT THANK YOU

As we close the pages of this journey toward better health and well-being, we stand at the cusp of a revolution in the way we understand and approach our bodies. Thanks to visionary voices in the health and wellness industry, the narrative has shifted—from relying on outdated paradigms to embracing science-backed, holistic practices that empower individuals to make informed, lasting changes.

From **Dr. Eric Berg**, who has redefined the way we view ketosis and intermittent fasting, offering life-changing advice to those seeking to optimize their metabolism, to **Dr. Mark Hyman**, a pioneer in functional medicine, whose deep understanding of nutrition and the power of personalized care has touched millions, the world is awakening to the profound impact of nutrition and lifestyle on overall health.

Rujuta Diwekar and **Prashant Desai**, two powerful voices in the wellness world who seamlessly blend the wisdom of tradition with the science of modern health, offering a holistic approach to nourishment and fitness. Their philosophies are rooted in the ancient practices that have stood the test of time, yet they are firmly grounded in the present, ensuring relevance in today's fast-paced world.

We are also fortunate to have **Dr. Palaniappan Manickam (Dr. Pal)**, a brilliant gastroenterologist, educating us on the importance of digestive health and its connection to vitality. Through his insightful teachings, he's igniting a movement of awareness around the gut-brain connection, empowering individuals to prioritize gut health as a cornerstone of wellness.

Ryan Fernando, an expert in sports nutrition, has shown us that health isn't just about looking good—it's about fueling our bodies to reach their highest potential. His wisdom in balancing fitness, nutrition, and mental resilience has transformed the lives of countless people.

Glucose Goddess, Jessie Inchauspé, has introduced us to the often-overlooked impact of blood sugar on health. Her empowering insights into glucose management are revolutionizing how we approach energy, mood, and overall longevity.

Each of these remarkable individuals has a unique specialization, but their collective message is clear: **Awareness** is the first step toward change. By embracing the wisdom of these experts, we are not just transforming our own health—we are creating a ripple effect that will lead to a world where more people live longer, healthier, and more fulfilling lives.

We are now in an era where knowledge is at our fingertips, where social media influencers are not just voices of influence, but guides leading the way toward a healthier, more informed society. Their dedication to spreading the truth about wellness, the science behind it, and the power of small, sustainable changes is what will truly create lasting transformation.

Let us continue to learn, grow, and take action toward a better tomorrow, inspired by those who are boldly paving the way for a future where health isn't just a goal, but a way of life.

The journey doesn't end here—it's only just begun.

ABOUT THE AUTHOR

Dr. Alekya Bejgam is a STEM engineer, combining creativity and science to solve real-world problems. A national awardee for innovation in medical device technology.

Her journey of excellence began early, with achievements like securing a state rank in the Math Olympiad, best speaker award by Toastmasters International and winning several science competitions. Beyond science, Dr. Bejgam has a deep love for art and takes her culinary experiments as seriously as her research. A true foodie, she finds joy in exploring flavors while nurturing her creative and analytical sides.

With a heart for family, children, humor, and nature, she embraces life's beauty with warmth and curiosity. Her debut book, *Biohacks 101*, is crafted for dreamers and hustlers aiming to make a mark in the world. She believes a healthier life fuels brighter futures, empowering individuals to uplift everyone around them.

www.ingramcontent.com/pod-product-compliance
Lightning Source LLC
Chambersburg PA
CBHW051235130726
47988CB00001B/356